CORE CLINICAL CASES
Self-assessment for Medical Students
Book 1

Second edition

A Problem-based Learning Approach

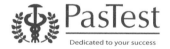

PasTest

Dedicated to your success

Dedication

To all those junior doctors subjected to MTAS (RIP), whether you are now at work or on the beaches down under!

CORE CLINICAL CASES
Self-assessment for Medical Students

Second edition

Andrew Sewart
Foundation Year 2 Doctor
Morecambe Bay Health Trust

Henriette van Ruiten
Foundation Year 2 Doctor
Morecambe Bay Health Trust

Edited by
Deborah Anne Wales MB ChB MRCP FRCA
Consultant Respiratory Physician
Nevill Hall Hospital
Abergavenny
Monmouthshire

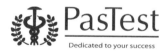

Parkgate Estate
Knutsford
Cheshire
WA16 8DX
Telephone: 01565 752000

Reprinted 2009

ISBN: 1 905635 338
ISBN: 978 1905635 337

A catalogue record for this book is available from the British Library.

PasTest Revision Books and Intensive Courses

PasTest has been established in the field of postgraduate medical education since 1972, providing revision books and intensive study courses for doctors preparing for their professional examinations. Books and courses are available for the following specialties:

MRCP Part 1 and Part 2, MRCPCH Part 1 and Part 2, MRCS, MRCOG, MRCGP, DRCOG, MRCPsych, DCH, FRCA and PLAB.

For further details contact:

PasTest, Freepost, Knutsford, Cheshire WA16 7BR

Tel: 01565 752000 Fax: 01565 650264

E-mail: enquiries@pastest.co.uk

Web site: www.pastest.co.uk

Typeset by Carnegie Book Production, Lancaster
Printed by CPI Antony Rowe, Chippenham, Wiltshire

CONTENTS

INTRODUCTION

We wrote the first edition of *Core Clinical Cases* when we were fourth year medical students. Three years have now passed of what has been a very steep, but thoroughly enjoyable, learning curve, and so this felt like the right time to update this book.

We have intentionally kept to the same format, namely a series of questions to prompt the student through the diagnosis and management of realistic clinical scenarios with the addition of radiographs, CT scans, ECGs and blood results for interpretation. This is quite simply to prepare you for when you start as Foundation Year doctors in a year or so time because these cases reflect real clinical scenarios with their management, following, where available, national clinical guidelines.

The main improvement on the first edition is the accompanying teaching notes, reflecting our growing clinical knowledge and experience, and as such we hope this will be used not only as a self-assessment book but also as a core reference book for your clinical attachments.

Finally, good luck in your future careers and we hope that you enjoy medicine as much as we do.

Andy and Henriette
Bouth
April 2007

CONTRIBUTORS

We would like the thank the following three doctors for all the time and effort that they spent reviewing the cases within their specialty and also for their help in writing new cases for this second edition.

James Galloway MBChB MRCP

Specialist Registrar in Rheumatology and General Medicine, North West Deanery

Spyridon I. Chouliaras MRCOG

Specialist Registrar in Obstetrics and Gynaecology, North West Deanery

Krasimir Atanasov

Staff Grade Paediatrician, Furness General Hospital, Morecambe Bay Health Trust

FOREWORD

It gave me great pleasure to be asked to review and write the foreword for this book for many reasons .....

I am delighted that two students have been so motivated by their learning that they have wanted to produce a *Problem Based Learning* book – and stuck with the project through to the end.

I am delighted that a book like this has been created – one that takes the problem that the patient presents with and uses that as a focus of learning. Not only is it sensible, as patients do not present with a label round their neck saying *'I have angina'* – or *'I have hypothyroidism'* – they present with the symptom that as clinicians we have to diagnose and manage, but more importantly, it reminds us that the reason for our learning is not a riddle to be solved but a patient for whose care we are responsible.

As a medical educator I am delighted that this book has been produced by and for students. It is one of the basic tenets of education that learning is driven by assessment. One of the difficulties about assessment is setting the standard and making it appropriate for the person being assessed – to have that done by and for students helps the student to focus their learning at the right level.

A S Garden
Head, Dept Medicine and Director,
Centre for Medical Education
Lancaster University

ABBREVIATIONS

A&E	accident and emergency
ABG	arterial blood gas
ACE	angiotensin-converting enzyme
ACS	acute coronary syndrome
ACTH	adrenocorticotrophic hormone
ADH	antidiuretic hormone
AF	atrial fibrillation
AFP	α-fetoprotein
AG	anion gap
AIDS	acquired immune deficiency syndrome
ALP	alkaline phosphatase
ALT	alanine transaminase
AMA	anti-mitochondrial antibody
ANA	anti-nuclear antibody
ANCA	anti-neutrophil cytoplasmic antibody
AP	anteroposterior or action potential
APTT	activated partial thromboplastin time
ARA	angiotension receptor antagonist
ARF	acute renal failure
5-ASA	5-aminosalicylic acid
AST	aspartate transaminase
ATN	acute tubular necrosis
AV	atrioventricular or arteriovenous
AVM	arteriovenous malformation
BE	base excess
BiPAP	bilevel positive airway pressure
BMI	body mass index
BNP	brain natriuretic peptide
BP	blood pressure
BPH	benign prostatic hypertrophy
BS	Bishop's score
CABG	coronary artery bypass graft
CBD	common bile duct
CCF	congestive cardiac (heart) failure
CFE	capital femoral epiphysis

CK	creatine kinase
CMV	cytomegalovirus
CN	cranial nerve
CNS	central nervous system
COC	combined oral contraceptive
COPD	chronic obstructive pulmonary disease
COX	cyclo-oxygenase
CPD	cephalopelvic disproportion
CRF	chronic renal failure
CRP	C-reactive protein
CSF	cerebrospinal fluid
CT	computed tomography
CTG	cardiotocography
CTPA	computed tomography pulmonary angiogram
CVA	cerebrovascular accident
CVD	cardiovascular disease
CVP	central venous pressure
CVS	chorionic villous sampling
DCT	direct Coombs' test
DDH	developmental dysplasia of the hip
DIC	disseminated intravascular coagulation
DIP	distal interphalangeal
DKA	diabetic ketoacidosis
DMARD	disease-modifying anti-rheumatic drug
DNA	deoxyribonucleic acid
DVT	deep vein thrombosis
EBV	Epstein–Barr virus
EC	emergency contraception
ECG	electrocardiogram
EDD	expected date of delivery
EMA	endomysial antibody
EPO	erythropoietin
ERCP	endoscopic retrograde cholangiopancreatography
ESR	erythrocyte sedimentation rate
ESRF	end-stage renal failure
ETT	exercise tolerance test
FBC	full blood count
FFP	fresh frozen plasma
FNA	fine-needle aspiration

FTT	failure to thrive
FT$_3$	free triiodothyronine
FT$_4$	free thyroxine
G&S	group and save
GBM	glomerular basement membrane
GBS	group B streptococcus
GCS	Glasgow Coma Scale
GFR	glomerular filtration rate
GGT	γ-glutamyl transferase
GI	gastrointestinal
GN	glomerulonephritis
GnRH	gonadotrophin-releasing hormone
GORD	gastro-oesophageal reflux disease
GTN	glyceryl trinitrate
GUM	genitourinary medicine
hCG	human chorionic gonadotrophin
hGH	human growth hormone
HIV	human immunodeficiency virus
HONK	hyperosmolar non-ketotic
HPOA	hypertrophic pulmonary osteoarthropathy
HR	heart rate
HRT	hormone replacement therapy
HSP	Henoch–Schönlein purpura
HSV	herpes simplex virus
HVS	high vaginal swab
IBD	inflammatory bowel disease
ICP	intracranial pressure
ICU	intensive care unit
IHD	ischaemic heart disease
INR	international normalised ratio
IU	international units
IUD	intrauterine device
IUGR	intrauterine growth retardation
IVDU	intravenous drug use(r)
JVP	jugular venous pressure
LAD	left anterior descending
LBBB	left bundle-branch block
LCPD	leg calf Perthes' disease
LDH	lactate dehydrogenase

LFTs	liver function tests
LH	luteinising hormone
LMP	last menstrual period
LMWH	low-molecular-weight heparin
LP	lumbar puncture
LV	left ventricular
LVF	left ventricular failure
LVH	left ventricular hypertrophy
MC&S	microscopy, culture and sensitivities
MCP	metacarpophalangeal
MCV	mean corpuscular volume
MI	myocardial infarction
MMSE	Mini-Mental State Examination
MRI	magnetic resonance imaging
NBM	nil by mouth
NGT	nasogastric tube
NGU	non-gonococcal urethritis
NICE	National Institute for Health and Clinical Excellence
NSAID	non-steroidal anti-inflammatory drug
NSTEMI	non-ST-elevation myocardial infarction
NT	nuchal translucency
NYHA	New York Heart Association
OGD	oesophagogastroduodenoscopy
OHSS	ovarian hyperstimulation syndrome
P_{CO_2}	partial pressure of carbon dioxide
P_{O_2}	partial pressure of oxygen
PA	posteroanterior
PAPP-A	pregnancy-associated plasma protein A
PBC	primary biliary cirrhosis
PCI	percutaneous coronary intervention
PCOS	polycystic ovarian syndrome
PCR	polymerase chain reaction
PE	pulmonary embolus
PEF	peak expiratory flow
PET	positron emission tomography
PID	pelvic inflammatory disease
PIE	pulmonary interstitial emphysema
PIP	proximal interphalangeal
PMR	polymyalgia rheumatica

PND	paroxysmal nocturnal dyspnoea
POP	progestogen-only pill
PPH	postpartum haemorrhage
PPI	proton pump inhibitor
PPROM	pre-term pre-labour rupture of membranes
PSA	prostate-specific antigen
PT	prothrombin time
PTCA	percutaneous transluminal coronary angioplasty
PTH	parathyroid hormone
PUD	peptic ulcer disease
PVD	peripheral vascular disease
RA	rheumatoid arthritis
RBC	red blood cells
RDS	respiratory distress syndrome
RF	rheumatoid factor
RSV	respiratory syncytial virus
RUQ	right upper quadrant
RV	right ventricular
RVF	right ventricular failure
SA	sinoatrial
Sao_2	arterial oxygen saturation
SCID	severe combined immune deficiency
SFE	slipped femoral epiphysis
SIADH	syndrome of inappropriate antidiuretic hormone secretion
SIRS	systemic inflammatory response syndrome
SLE	systemic lupus erythematosus
SMA	smooth muscle antibody
STEMI	ST-elevation myocardial infarction
STI	sexually transmitted infection
SVC	superior vena cava
SVT	supraventricular tachycardia
T_3	triiodothyronine
T_4	thyroxine
TB	tuberculosis
TBG	thyroxine-binding globulin
TC	total cholesterol
TED	thromboembolic deterrent
TENS	transcutaneous electrical nerve stimulation
TFTs	thyroid function tests

TIA	transient ischaemic attack
TNF-α	tumour necrosis factor alpha
tTG	tissue transglutaminase
TSH	thyroid-stimulating hormone
U&Es	urea and electrolytes
UC	ulcerative colitis
UPSI	unprotected sexual intercourse
UTI	urinary tract infection
VSD	ventricular septal defect
VT	ventricular tachycardia
WBC	white blood cell
WCC	white cell count

CARDIOVASCULAR
CASES: QUESTIONS

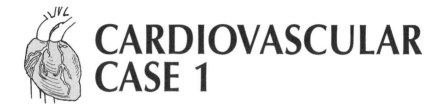

CARDIOVASCULAR CASE 1

James, a 68-year-old lifelong smoker, is brought into accident and emergency (A&E) by ambulance. He has a 45-minute history of central, crushing chest pain associated with nausea, dyspnoea and sweating. On cardiovascular examination, his blood pressure is 164/96 mmHg, heart rate 92 beats/min and regular; jugular venous pressure (JVP) is 4 cm above the sternal angle, heart sounds are normal and the chest is clear.

Q List six differential diagnoses　　　　　　　　**3 marks**

1.

2.

3.

4.

5.

6.

James's ECG is shown:

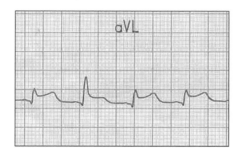

Q What is the abnormality?   1 mark

1. _____

This abnormality is seen in leads I, aVL and V5–6.

Q What is the most likely diagnosis?   2 marks

1. _____

Q What other ECG changes may be expected to develop?   1 mark

1. _____

2. _____

Q What is your immediate management?   3 marks

1. _____

2. _____

3. _____

4. _____

5. _____

6. _____

The patient undergoes thrombolysis within 4 hours.

Q List two ECG indications for thrombolysis   2 marks

1. _____

2. _____

Q Name three absolute contraindications for thrombolysis   3 marks

1. _____

2. _____

3. _____

Q List five complications of myocardial infarction   5 marks

1. _____

2. _____

3. _____

4. _____

5. _____

James is discharged 5 days later with no complications.

Q What advice, treatment and investigations would you recommend
to reduce his risk of a similar episode?   5 marks

1. _____

2. _____

3. _____

4. _____

5. _____

Total: 25 marks

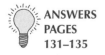
ANSWERS
PAGES
131–135

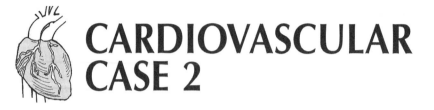

CARDIOVASCULAR CASE 2

Sarah, a 77-year-old woman, attends A&E complaining of palpitations. Her ECG is shown below.

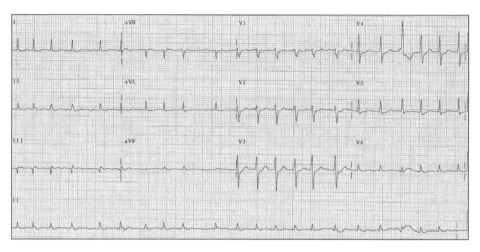

Q What does the ECG show? 2 marks

1.

Q List six causes of this rhythm 3 marks

1.

2.

3.

4.

5.

6.

Q What six other investigations would you do?   3 marks

1.

2.

3.

4.

5.

6.

Q What two drugs may be used for rate control?   2 marks

1.

2.

Q What two methods may be used to attempt cardioversion?   2 marks

1.

2.

Q What two drugs may be used for rhythm control?   2 marks

1.

2.

Q What class of anti-arrhythmic is amiodarone in?   2 marks

1.

Q List three side effects of amiodarone   3 marks

1.

2.

3.

Q Name three complications if her rhythm is not appropriately
   treated   3 marks

1.

2.

3.

Q What drug is used for anticoagulation, how is it monitored and what is the
   target range?   3 marks

1.

2.

3.

Total   25 marks

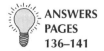
ANSWERS
PAGES
136–141

CARDIOVASCULAR CASE 3

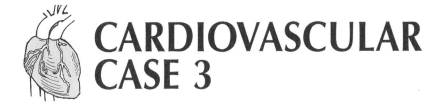

David, a 51-year-old man, has attended his GP for his third blood pressure measurement; his three readings are 167/96, 162/104 and 174/104.

Q **Define the systolic/diastolic ranges for mild (phase 1), moderate (phase 2) and severe (phase 3) hypertension** 3 marks

1. Mild:

2. Moderate:

3. Severe:

You request an ECG, shown below:

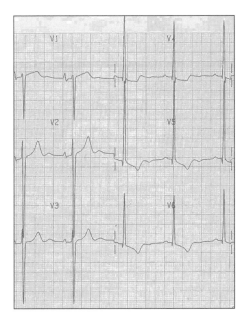

Q What does his ECG show? 1 mark

1.

Q Why is this important with regard to hypertension? 1 mark

1.

Q List four additional initial investigations that you would do 4 marks

1.

2.

3.

4.

Q List three causes of secondary hypertension 3 marks

1.

2.

3.

Q List three reasons when you would consider referring a hypertensive patient for specialist care 3 marks

1.

2.

3.

You determine that David's blood pressure needs to be treated.

Cardiovascular

Q **What three lifestyle changes would you recommend?** 3 marks

1.

2.

3.

Q **What are the first-line antihypertensives?** 3 marks

1.

2.

3.

You prescribe David an angiotensin-converting enzyme (ACE) inhibitor.

Q **What two electrolyte abnormalities may ACE inhibitors cause?** 2 marks

1.

2.

Q **Name four complications if David's hypertension is not treated** 2 marks

1.

2.

3.

4.

Total 25 marks

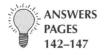

**ANSWERS
PAGES
142–147**

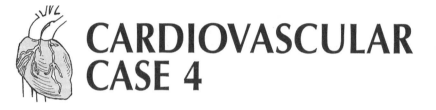

CARDIOVASCULAR CASE 4

Tim, a 60-year-old man, visits his GP complaining of recent episodes of central chest tightness on exertion. These settle on rest and last no longer than 5–10 minutes. There is nothing of note in his past medical history. Cardiovascular examination is normal.

Q **The clinical suspicion is of angina pectoris. What are the main risk factors for ischaemic heart disease (IHD)?**   **5 marks**

1.

2.

3.

4.

5.

All of Tim's blood tests are normal except a fasting total cholesterol (TC) of 7.2 mmol/L.

Q **What is the recommended upper limit for fasting TC in the secondary prevention of IHD?**   **2 marks**

1.

Tim is prescribed a statin by his GP.

Q What blood test must you request before prescribing a statin and what advice must you give to patients on statin therapy **4 marks**

1.

2.

Tim's resting ECG is normal. His GP arranges an appointment as an outpatient for an exercise tolerance test (ETT) in order to diagnose angina.

Q Indicate whether each of the following exercise ECG represents a negative or positive ETT **3 marks**

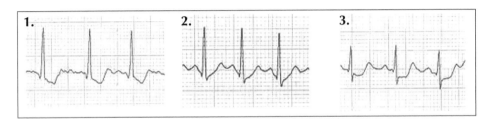

1. ECG 1:

2. ECG 2:

3. ECG 3:

Tim's exercise tolerance test is strongly positive and a diagnosis of angina is made. His cardiologist prescribes 75 mg aspirin once daily, addresses his modifiable risk factors and places him on the waiting list for coronary angiography.

Q List four drugs that may be prescribed to control angina **4 marks**

1.

2.

TVO7609

3.

4.

Three months later Tim undergoes angiography, which shows severe stenosis of one of his coronary arteries.

Q What two procedures are available to treat the stenosed artery?   **2 marks**

1.

2.

Total   **20 marks**

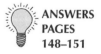

ANSWERS
PAGES
148–151

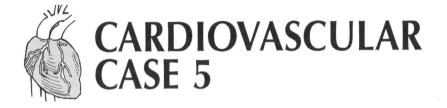

CARDIOVASCULAR CASE 5

John, a 72-year-old man, is referred by his GP to cardiac outpatients complaining of a 3-month history of progressive breathlessness. He is now breathless even when doing simple tasks around the home, such as dressing. He is currently prescribed medications for his hypertension and inflammatory arthritis.

Q List four non-cardiac causes of gradually progressive dyspnoea   2 marks

1.

2.

3.

4.

Q From the history above classify his heart failure according to the New York Heart Association (NYHA) criteria   2 marks

1.

Q List four symptoms suggestive of left ventricular failure (LVF)   2 marks

1.

2.

3.

4.

15

Q **What hormone is significantly raised in heart failure?**　　　1 mark

1.

Q **What key investigation would you do to confirm heart failure?**　　2 marks

1.

John is diagnosed with congestive cardiac failure.

John's posteroanterior (PA) chest radiograph is shown.

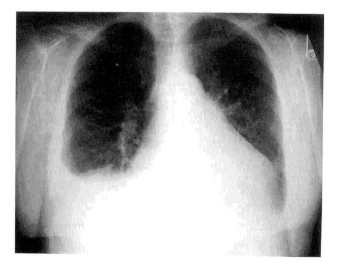

Q **List two features seen on the chest radiograph**　　　2 marks

1.

2.

Q **List four causes of LVF**　　　4 marks

1.

2.

3.

4.

John is being treated for both hypertension and inflammatory arthritis with the following medications: aspirin, verapamil, carvedilol, methotrexate and diclofenac.

Q **Which of these drugs should be avoided now that a diagnosis of heart failure has been made?** 2 marks

1.

2.

John's cardiologist commences him on an ACE inhibitor and furosemide.

Q **List three electrolyte abnormalities caused by furosemide** 3 marks

1.

2.

3.

Total 20 marks

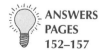

ANSWERS
PAGES
152–157

ENDOCRINOLOGY CASES: QUESTIONS

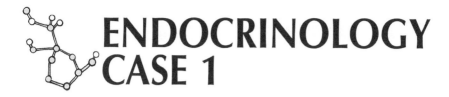

ENDOCRINOLOGY
CASE 1

Gloria, a 38-year-old woman, is referred by her GP to an endocrinologist with symptoms of thyrotoxicosis.

Q Name six symptoms that Gloria may be complaining of 3 marks

1.

2.

3.

4.

5.

6.

On examination she is in sinus tachycardia, and has a fine tremor and bulging eyes (exophthalmos).

Q List four signs specific to Graves' disease 2 marks

1.

2.

3.

4.

Q **What is the underlying cause of Graves' disease?**   2 marks

1.

Bloods are taken for thyroid function tests (TFTs), as shown in the table.

Q **Indicate (↑, ↓ or ↔) where marked '?' for the expected changes**   3 marks

Hormone	Normal range	Hyperthyroidism
TSH (mU/L)	0.5–5.7	?
Total T$_4$ (nmol/L)	70–140	?
Total T$_3$ (nmol/L)	1.2–3.0	?

T$_3$, triiodothyronine; T$_4$, thyroxine; TSH, thyroid-stimulating hormone.

Gloria's symptoms are treated with β blockers and her hyperthyroidism by 'block-and-replace' regimen with carbimazole and thyroxine.

Q **Give one short-term and one long-term complication if her hyperthyroidism is untreated**   2 marks

1. **Short-term complication:**

2. **Long-term complication:**

Q **Give four indications for thyroidectomy in Gloria**   2 marks

1.

2.

3.

4.

22

Q Give four complications of surgery   2 marks

1.

2.

3.

4.

On cessation of the 'block-and-replace' regimen Gloria remains hyperthyroid. She is subsequently treated with radioactive iodine, which initially renders her euthyroid, although eventually it leaves her hypothyroid.

Q List four other causes of hypothyroidism   4 marks

1.

2.

3.

4.

Total   **20 marks**

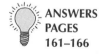

ANSWERS
PAGES
161–166

ENDOCRINOLOGY CASE 2

Jenny, a 21-year-old woman with type 1 diabetes, is seen by her GP after a 2-day history of nausea and vomiting; now she is complaining of abdominal pain. Urine dipstick showed glycosuria and ketonuria, and she is admitted to the medical assessment unit. On examination her GCS (Glasgow Coma Score) is 15/15, heart rate (HR) 120/min, abdomen tender throughout, and she is hyperventilating and appears to be dehydrated.

Q How is diabetic ketoacidosis (DKA) diagnosed biochemically? 3 marks

1.

2.

3.

Q List three causes of DKA 3 marks

1.

2.

3.

Jenny is diagnosed with DKA. Her arterial blood gases (ABGs) are shown in the table.

Q Indicate (↑, ↓ or ↔) where marked '?' for the expected changes 4 marks

	Normal range	Jenny's ABGs
pH	7.35–7.45	?
P_{O_2} (kPa)	10–12	11
P_{CO_2} (kPa)	4.7–6	?
HCO_3^- (mmol/L)	22–28	?
Base excess or BE (mmol/L)	±2	–9
Anion gap	10–18	?

Q How do you calculate the anion gap? 1 mark

1.

Q List three causes of metabolic acidosis with an *increased* anion gap 3 marks

1.

2.

3.

Jenny is successfully treated with intravenous fluids and intravenous insulin.

Q List three complications of this treatment 3 marks

1.

2.

3.

Once stabilised Jenny is referred to the diabetic nurse specialist for advice on the management of her diabetes.

Q List four 'illness rules' that you would give Jenny   2 marks

1.

2.

3.

4.

Q List four warning signs of hypoglycaemia   2 marks

1.

2.

3.

4.

Q What two coexisting conditions should you screen for in Jenny?   2 marks

1.

2.

Q List two challenges facing Jenny   2 marks

1.

2.

Total   25 marks

ANSWERS
PAGES
167–172

GASTROINTESTINAL
CASES: QUESTIONS

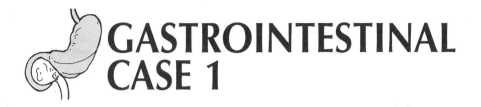

GASTROINTESTINAL CASE 1

*Henry, a 58-year-old man, presents to accident and emergency
(A&E) with a 1-hour history of haematemesis, including a severe
episode in the ambulance. On examination his BP is 86/44 mmHg,
he is cold peripherally and his pulse is 110 beats/min.*

Q List six causes of haematemesis   3 marks

1.

2.

3.

4.

5.

6.

Q What is your immediate management?   3 marks

1.

2.

3.

Q What three brief questions would you ask?   3 marks

1.

2.

3.

Q What four blood tests would you request?   2 marks

1.

2.

3.

4.

Henry undergoes emergency endoscopy, which diagnoses an actively bleeding gastric ulcer; this is successfully treated by an injection of epinephrine (adrenaline).

Q What factors are used to assess Henry's risk of re-bleeding?   4 marks

1.

2.

3.

4.

Q List four signs of a re-bleed while on the ward   2 marks

1.

2.

3.

4.

Henry's rapid urease text on endoscopy confirms Helicobacter pylori *infection, and the endoscopist recommends triple therapy for eradication and avoiding non-steroidal anti-inflammatory drugs (NSAIDs).*

Q What does this regimen involve? 1 mark

1.

Q Name two drugs used to reduce gastrointestinal (GI) side effects of NSAIDs 2 marks

1.

2.

Total 20 marks

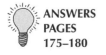
Gastrointestinal

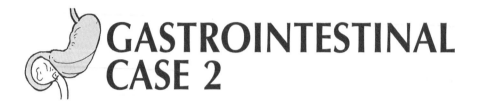

GASTROINTESTINAL CASE 2

Rod, a 48-year-old man, is admitted to the medical assessment unit complaining of malaise and anorexia. On examination he is jaundiced with signs of chronic liver disease.

Q List four risk factors for jaundice that you would enquire about in the *social* history 2 marks

1.

2.

3.

4.

Q List three *abdominal* signs of chronic liver disease 3 marks

1.

2.

3.

Several blood tests are requested to assess the severity of Rod's liver failure.

Q Name two blood tests used to assess liver synthetic function 2 marks

1.

2. _____

Abdominal ultrasonography reports cirrhotic changes in the liver (later confirmed on liver biopsy) with gross ascites.

Q In the absence of obvious risk factors list six blood tests that you would request to identify the cause of Rod's liver cirrhosis   3 marks

1. _____

2. _____

3. _____

4. _____

5. _____

6. _____

It is apparent from Rod's social history that the cause of his liver failure is alcoholic liver disease and he is given intravenous thiamine and started on a chlordiazepoxide-reducing regimen.

Q Why do we give thiamine to people with alcohol problems?   1 mark

1. _____

Q How would you treat Rod's ascites?   3 marks

1. _____

2. _____

3. _____

Gastrointestinal

Several days later Rod starts to deteriorate, complaining of severe abdominal pain. On examination his abdomen is very tender with guarding, and he is pyrexial.

Q What is the likely complication?　　　　　　　　2 marks

1.

Q How would you confirm your diagnosis?　　　　　　1 mark

1.

Q List three additional complications of liver cirrhosis　　3 marks

1.

2.

3.

Total　　　　　　　　　　　　　　　　　　**20 marks**

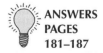ANSWERS
PAGES
181–187

Gastrointestinal

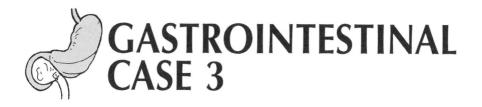# GASTROINTESTINAL CASE 3

Dennis, a 64-year-old man, is admitted to the surgical assessment unit with a history of severe epigastric pain, radiating to his back, of several hours associated with nausea and vomiting. His serum amylase is reported as 670 U/mL (normal range 0–180 U/mL), confirming a diagnosis of acute pancreatitis.

Q List eight criteria used to assess the severity of pancreatitis   **4 marks**

1.

2.

3.

4.

5.

6.

7.

8.

Q List three causes of acute pancreatitis   **3 marks**

1.

2.

3.

Dennis is kept nil by mouth (NBM), and given high-flow oxygen therapy and aggressive fluid replacement. A urinary catheter is inserted to monitor his urine output.

Q In fluid replacement, what minimum hourly urinary output do you aim for?

1 mark

1.

Dennis undergoes an abdominal ultrasound scan, which shows gallbladder stones with their acoustic shadows.

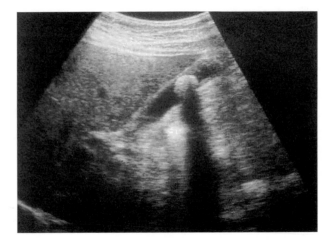

Q Name six additional complications of gallstones
3 marks

1.

2.

3.

4.

5.

6.

Q **What is the recommended procedure within the first 72 hours?** 2 marks

1.

Dennis undergoes a cholecystectomy before discharge.

Q **List two advantages each of laparoscopic and open cholecystectomy** 4 marks

1. Laparoscopic:

2. Open:

Q **Give three complications of cholecystectomy** 3 marks

1.

2.

3.

Total 20 marks

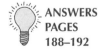

ANSWERS
PAGES
188–192

Gastrointestinal

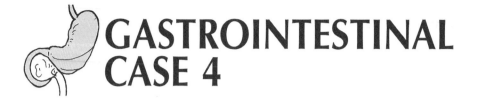

GASTROINTESTINAL CASE 4

Annie, a 25-year-old woman, presents with a 4-week history of diarrhoea with some mucus and blood mixed in her stool. She also complains of general abdominal discomfort, malaise and weight loss.

Q List four causes of bloody diarrhoea   **4 marks**

1.

2.

3.

4.

Q Why would you do a plain abdominal radiograph in an acute attack of ulcerative colitis?   **2 marks**

1.

2.

Annie is given a phosphate enema and undergoes a sigmoidoscopy, which reveals a superficial continuous inflammation of the rectum. The mucosa looks reddened and inflamed, consistent with ulcerative colitis (UC).

Q List four pathological differences between UC and Crohn's disease   4 marks

1.

2.

3.

4.

Q List four extraintestinal manifestations of inflammatory bowel disease (IBD)   2 marks

1.

2.

3.

4.

Q List six features used to assess the severity of UC   3 marks

1.

2.

3.

4.

5.

6.

Annie is treated with oral and rectal steroids and responds well to treatment.

Q **What class of drug is prescribed to maintain remission in UC?**   **2 marks**

1.

Q **Give three complications of ulcerative colitis**   **3 marks**

1.

2.

3.

Total   **20 marks**

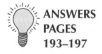
ANSWERS
PAGES
193–197

Gastrointestinal

NEUROLOGY CASES: QUESTIONS

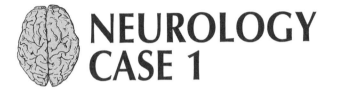

NEUROLOGY
CASE 1

George, a 72-year-old man on treatment for hypertension, is admitted with a stroke. Examination reveals weakness, sensory loss and homonymous hemianopia on the affected side.

Q List two visual symptoms that George might be complaining of   **2 marks**

1.

2.

Q Name two sensory modalities carried in the posterior column   **2 marks**

1.

2.

Q Name four cardiac conditions that may cause an embolic stroke   **4 marks**

1.

2.

3.

4.

Q List six features associated with a lesion to the vertebrobasilar territory   **3 marks**

1.

2. _____

3. _____

4. _____

5. _____

6. _____

George undergoes a number of investigations including computed tomography (CT) of the brain.

George's brain CT scan is shown.

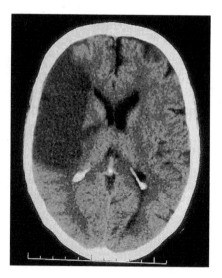

Q **Is George's stroke the result of an infarction or a haemorrhage?**   1 mark

1. _____

Q **What cerebral artery is affected?**   2 marks

1. _____

Q **List six additional investigations that you might consider, briefly explaining why** 3 marks

1.

2.

3.

4.

5.

6.

George is transferred to the stroke ward for rehabilitation where, over the following weeks, he makes good progress.

Q **Name six health professionals involved in George's rehabilitation** 3 marks

1.

2.

3.

4.

5.

6.

Total 20 marks

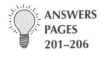
ANSWERS PAGES 201–206

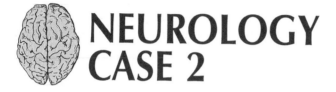

NEUROLOGY CASE 2

Ethel, an 82-year-old widow, is admitted after her carer found her that morning still in bed and more confused than normal.

Q List five causes of acute confusion (delirium)   **5 marks**

1.

2.

3.

4.

5.

On examination she has a Glasgow Coma Score (GCS) of 11/15, temperature 38.5°C, BP 116/64 mmHg, heart rate (HR) 90 regular, respiratory rate 28/min and pulse oximetry 87 per cent, and there is bronchial breathing at her right lung base.

Q List three non-invasive investigations that you would do   **3 marks**

1.

2.

3.

Ethel's blood test results are shown in the table.

Variable	Value	Normal range	Variable	Value	Normal range	Variable	Value	Normal range
Hb (g/dL)	14.8	11.5–16	Sodium (mmol/L)	151	135–145	pH	7.41	7.35–7.45
MCV (fL)	84	76–96	Potassium (mmol/L)	4.1	3.5–5	Po_2 (kPa)	7.6	> 10.6
WCC (neutrophilia) ($\times 10^9$/L)	18	4–11	Urea (mmol/L)	16	2.5–6.7	PCo_2 (kPa)	5.1	4.7–6
Platelets ($\times 10^9$/L)	331	150–400	Creatinine (µmol/L)	211	70–120	HCO_3^- (mmol/L)	24	22–28
CRP (mg/L)	143	< 10	Albumin (g/L)	24	35–50	BE (mmol/L)	–1.2	±2
Glucose (mmol/L)	22.7	4–6	Calcium (mmol/L)	1.93				
			Adjusted calcium	N/A	2.12–2.65			

BE, base excess; CRP, C-reactive protein; MCV, mean corpuscular volume; WCC, white cell count.

Q Calculate Ethel's adjusted calcium   1 mark

1.

Q List five diagnoses inferred from these blood results   5 marks

1.

2.

3.

4.

5.

A diagnosis of pneumonia is made and Ethel is successfully treated with oxygen therapy, intravenous antibiotics, sliding scale insulin and intravenous fluids. Before discharge her underlying dementia is assessed and she records a Mini-Mental State Examination (MMSE) score of 18.

Q **What MMSE score supports a diagnosis of dementia?**   1 mark

1.

Q **What are the two most common causes of dementia?**   1 mark

1.

2.

Q **List four blood tests that you would do to exclude treatable causes of dementia**   4 marks

1.

2.

3.

4.

Total   20 marks

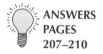

ANSWERS
PAGES
207–210

NEUROLOGY CASE 3

Matthew, an 18-year-old student, is found by his flatmates complaining of headache, stiff neck and photophobia. Worried that he may have meningitis, they rush him straight to the accident and emergency department (A&E).

Q Name two signs associated with meningeal irritation   **2 marks**

1.

2.

Before a lumbar puncture (LP) is performed Matthew is examined to exclude raised intracranial pressure.

Q List six signs suggesting raised ICP   **6 marks**

1.

2.

3.

4.

5.

6.

Q Give two contraindications (other than raised ICP) to LP 2 marks

1.

2.

There are no signs of raised ICP and an LP is performed.

Q Indicate (↑, → or ↓) where marked '?' for the expected cerebrospinal fluid (CSF) changes in bacterial meningitis 3 marks

	Normal	Bacterial meningitis
Appearance	Clear	Turbid
WCC (/mm³)	≤ 5 (no neutrophils)	?
Protein (g/L)	0.2–0.4	?
Glucose (% plasma glucose)	> 50	?

Matthew is diagnosed with meningococcal meningitis, his CSF Gram stain confirming Neisseria meningitidis.

Q What colour does *Neisseria meningitidis* Gram stain? 1 mark

1.

Q List four complications of bacterial meningitis 4 marks

1.

2.

3.

4.

Neurology

Q **What prophylaxis do you give to contacts of Matthew and what do you warn them about?** 2 marks

1. _____

2. _____

Total **20 marks**

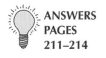

ANSWERS
PAGES
211–214

OBSTETRICS AND GYNAECOLOGY CASES: QUESTIONS

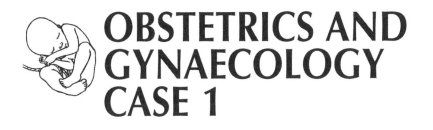

OBSTETRICS AND GYNAECOLOGY CASE 1

Katie, who is 28 weeks into her first pregnancy, suddenly experiences a gush of fluid vaginally in the absence of any uterine contractions. Cardiotocography (CTG) is normal and ultrasonography shows reduced residual amniotic fluid. A speculum examination is performed, which reveals a closed cervix and pooling of fluid in the posterior vaginal fornix.

Q List four causes of pre-term pre-labour rupture of membranes (PPROM)   2 marks

1.

2.

3.

4.

Q From what common vaginal organism is Katie's baby at risk?   1 mark

1.

Q List two treatments to decrease perinatal complications   2 marks

1.

2.

On examination, Katie's temperature is 38°C, heart rate 92 beats/min and she has raised inflammatory markers. As a result of the risks of maternal and fetal infection, it is decided to induce labour. Her cervix is assessed using Bishop's score.

Q List four features used to assess Bishop's score　　　　**2 marks**

1.

2.

3.

4.

Q What Bishop's score is considered ripe for induction?　　　　**1 mark**

1.

Q What is used to make the cervix ripe for induction?　　　　**1 mark**

1.

Katie's contractions are inefficient so she is started with an infusion of oxytocin.

Q List two potential complications of using oxytocin in Katie　　**2 marks**

1.

2.

Obstetrics

Katie delivers a girl called Emma weighing 1.1 kg. At 1 minute of life Emma's extremities are bluish, her limbs flaccid, her breathing irregular, she grimaces when the soles of her feet are stimulated and her heart rate is 82 beats/min.

Q **Calculate Emma's 1-minute Apgar score**   **2 marks**

1. _____

Within an hour of birth Emma starts developing signs of respiratory distress. She is intubated by the neonatologist, artificial surfactant is instilled and she is artificially ventilated.

Q **List four pulmonary causes of respiratory distress in a neonate**   **2 marks**

1. _____

2. _____

3. _____

4. _____

Q **List two complications of artificially ventilating Emma**   **2 marks**

1. _____

2. _____

Obstetrics

57

Emma's chest radiograph is shown.

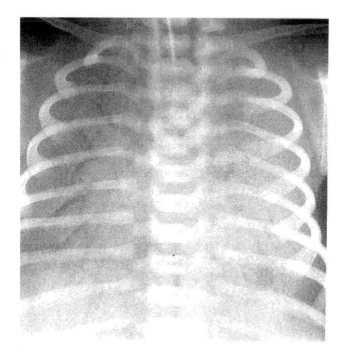

Q Describe three abnormalities on the chest radiograph　　　　**3 marks**

1.

2.

3.

Total　　　　**20 marks**

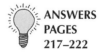
ANSWERS
PAGES
217–222

Obstetrics

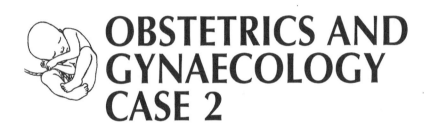

OBSTETRICS AND GYNAECOLOGY CASE 2

Paul and Julie (both aged 33 years) visit their GP after 2 years of being unable to conceive. A full history is taken from both. Julie's gynaecological history reveals irregular periods.

Q What general advice would you give to couples trying to get pregnant?   **2 marks**

1.

2.

3.

4.

Q List four points in the full history suggestive of tubal dysfunction   **4 marks**

1.

2.

3.

4.

As an initial assessment the GP organises a semen analysis for Paul and requests a number of blood tests from Julie.

Q List three variables measured in semen analysis   3 marks

1.

2.

3.

The results come back confirming normal semen analysis. Julie's blood results are shown in the table.

LH (day 2)	18 U/L (normal range 3–16)
FSH (day 2)	6 U/L (normal range 2–8)
Progesterone (day 21 – mid-luteal)	8 nmol/L

LH, luteinising hormone; FSH, follicle-stimulating hormone.

Q What is a normal day 21 progesterone concentration?   1 mark

1.

Q Give two explanations for Julie's progesterone concentration   2 marks

1.

2.

Q What might an FSH much greater than 10 U/L on day 2 suggest?   1 mark

1.

Q What is your likely diagnosis?   1 mark

1.

Obstetrics

Q List three clinical features that Julie might have 3 marks

1.

2.

3.

Julie is referred to her local infertility clinic. She has a hysterosalpingogram that is normal. Her infertility is treated with clomifene.

Q List three complications associated with this treatment 3 marks

1.

2.

3.

Total 20 marks

Obstetrics

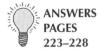

ANSWERS
PAGES
223–228

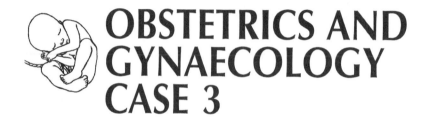

OBSTETRICS AND GYNAECOLOGY CASE 3

Debbie, aged 26 years, is out walking when her waters break. She is rushed to the labour ward by her husband Gerald, complaining of regular painful contractions every 10 minutes.

Q List four questions that you would ask　　　　　**2 marks**

1.

2.

3.

4.

On obstetric palpation her fundal height corresponds to her dates (she is 39 weeks' pregnant with her first child), the lie is longitudinal, the presentation cephalic and the fetal head engaged. On vaginal examination the position is left occipitoanterior and the cervix is 4 cm dilated.

Q List six *maternal* observations recorded on the partogram　　　**3 marks**

1.

2.

3.

4.

5.

6.

Debbie's contractions become progressively more frequent and painful. Three hours later her cervical dilatation is reassessed and plotted on the partogram, demonstrating that Debbie's labour is progressing satisfactorily.

Q Give two examples each of non-pharmacological and pharmacological methods of pain relief   **2 marks**

1. Non-pharmacological:

2. Pharmacological:

Q By how many centimetres should the cervix be dilated by now?   **1 mark**

1.

Q List four causes of failure to progress in the first stage of labour   **2 marks**

1.

2.

3.

4.

During labour, Debbie's baby is intermittently monitored by cardiotocography CTG to assess whether her baby is distressed.

Q What four components are used to interpret a CTG? 2 marks

1.

2.

3.

4.

Q List four sequential stages in the passage of the fetus through the birth canal leading up to the delivery of the shoulders 4 marks

1.

2.

3.

4.

Debbie delivers a pink and healthy boy called Alex who cries immediately.

Q List four steps in your immediate management of Alex 2 marks

1.

2.

3.

4.

As Alex is born, Debbie is given intramuscular Syntometrine (oxytocin with ergometrine). Following the birth the placenta is removed by controlled cord traction and inspected for completeness.

Q Give two non-pharmacological techniques for reducing postpartum haemorrhage (PPH)   **1 mark**

1. _____

2. _____

Q Name two drugs that are used in the management of PPH   **1 mark**

1. _____

2. _____

Total   **20 marks**

Obstetrics

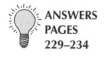

ANSWERS PAGES 229–234

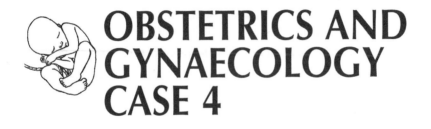

OBSTETRICS AND GYNAECOLOGY CASE 4

Sue and her husband Peter are both delighted to discover that Sue is pregnant for the first time. Sue is now 10 weeks' pregnant (her last menstrual period [LMP] was 15 July and her cycle is normally a regular 28 days) and she attends the antenatal clinic for her booking visit.

Q When is Sue's expected date of delivery (EDD) according to Naegele's rule?　　　　1 mark

1. _____

Q List six blood tests you would offer　　　　3 marks

1. _____

2. _____

3. _____

4. _____

5. _____

6. _____

4.

5.

6.

7.

8 .

Nothing in her history contraindicates the pill. She is prescribed a 3-month supply of a COC and advised on its side effects.

Q Name six *minor* side effects that Ageeth may experience   3 marks

1.

2.

3.

4.

5.

6.

Q List six pieces of additional advice that you would give Ageeth   3 marks

1.

2.

3.

4.

Obstetrics

5. _____

6. _____

Several months later Ageeth attends her genitourinary medicine (GUM) clinic complaining of an offensive vaginal discharge.

Q List four additional clinical features that would suggest pelvic inflammatory disease (PID)   2 marks

1. _____

2. _____

3. _____

4. _____

Q What six questions would you ask in the sexual history?   3 marks

1. _____

2. _____

3. _____

4. _____

5. _____

6. _____

Obstetrics

Q List three causes of vaginal discharge   3 marks

1.

2.

3.

Endocervical and high vaginal swabs are taken. Microscopy reveals pink Gram-stained diplococci.

Q What is the likely cause of her vaginal discharge?   1 mark

1.

Q List four additional tests that you would offer Ageeth   2 marks

1.

2.

3.

4.

Total   **25 marks**

Obstetrics

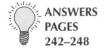

ANSWERS PAGES 242–248

PAEDIATRIC CASES: QUESTIONS

Q List four examples of dietary advice that you would give Sue   2 marks

1.

2.

3.

4.

Q List eight common minor symptoms of pregnancy that Sue may experience   4 marks

1.

2.

3.

4.

5.

6.

7.

8.

As a result of her age Sue has an increased risk of chromosomal abnormalities including Down's syndrome (her risk is 1:338).

Q Name two markers measured to screen for trisomy 21   2 marks

1.

2.

Q List six symptoms associated with pre-eclampsia　　　　3 marks

1.

2.

3.

4.

5.

6.

Q What four investigations would you do in pre-eclampsia?　　2 marks

1.

2.

3.

4.

At 28 weeks Sue attends the antenatal clinic for her regular antenatal care. On obstetric examination the midwife finds that the fundal height is 24 cm.

Q Give four reasons why Sue may be small for dates　　　2 marks

1.

2.

3.

4.

Q List six causes of intrauterine growth retardation (IUGR)   3 marks

1.

2.

3.

4.

5.

6.

Q List six topics that you want to discuss with Sue in her third
trimester   3 marks

1.

2.

3.

4.

5.

6.

Total   25 marks

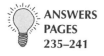
ANSWERS
PAGES
235–241

Obstetrics

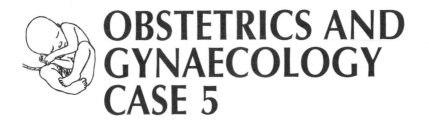

OBSTETRICS AND GYNAECOLOGY CASE 5

Ageeth, a 26-year-old-woman, visits her GP on Monday requesting emergency contraception. She recently started a new relationship and had unprotected sexual intercourse on Saturday night. She is on day 9 of her 28-day cycle.

Q What would you advise Ageeth?   2 marks

1.

2.

She opts for hormonal emergency contraception and chooses the pill for future contraception.

Q Describe two contraceptive mechanisms of combined oral contraceptives (COCs)   2 marks

1.

2.

Q List eight *absolute* contraindications to COCs   4 marks

1.

2.

3.

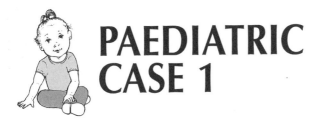

PAEDIATRIC CASE 1

Chelsea, aged 3 months, is brought into the accident and emergency department (A&E) by her parents with a 2-day history of feeding difficulties preceded by coryzal symptoms. On examination she is pyrexial and appears dehydrated. Furthermore she has signs of respiratory distress with a widespread expiratory wheeze; her arterial oxygen saturation (Sao_2; on air) is 90 per cent.

Q Give six causes of wheezing in an infant   3 marks

1.

2.

3.

4.

5.

6.

Q List six signs of respiratory distress in an infant   3 marks

1.

2.

3.

4.

5.

6.

Q **What are the normal heart and respiratory rates in infants?**   2 marks

1. Heart rate:

2. Respiratory rate:

Q **List eight signs indicating dehydration in an infant**   2 marks

1.

2.

3.

4.

5.

6.

7.

8.

Q **How are the maintenance fluid requirements for a child calculated?** 2 marks

1.

Chelsea is diagnosed with bronchiolitis and is admitted on to the ward and barrier nursed to prevent spread.

Paediatrics

Q What are the four cardinal signs of bronchiolitis? 2 marks

1.

2.

3.

4.

Q List four types of patient at risk of bronchiolitis 2 marks

1.

2.

3.

4.

Q What is the common cause of bronchiolitis and how is it detected? 2 marks

1.

2.

Q How would you manage Chelsea? 3 marks

1.

2.

3.

Q What is the prophylactic antibody for respiratory syncytial virus (RSV) 2 marks

1.

Q How would you monitor the effectiveness of treatment? 2 marks

1.

2.

3.

4.

Total 25 marks

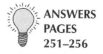

ANSWERS
PAGES
251–256

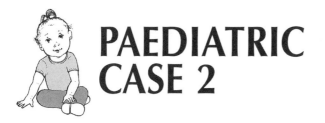

PAEDIATRIC CASE 2

James, aged 3 years, is referred to the paediatric outpatient clinic because of poor weight gain over the last 6 months. He was born at full term weighing 3.2 kg. However, over the last 6 months his mum says that he has become irritable, his abdomen seems distended and he has lots of liquid stools that are foul smelling and difficult to flush. On examination James is pale and his abdomen protrudes. There is wasting of his muscles (especially buttocks) and his ankles seem swollen.

Q **Define failure to thrive**   2 marks

1.

Q **List four non-organic causes of failure to thrive**   4 marks

1.

2.

3.

4.

Q **What is the mechanism of James's diarrhoea?**   1 mark

1.

Q What is the underlying cause of James's ankle oedema?   2 marks

1. _____

As part of his investigations James is screened for coeliac disease.

Q What is the most sensitive and specific screening test for coeliac disease?   1 mark

1. _____

James's screening test is positive and he is referred for a jejunal biopsy, which subsequently confirms coeliac disease.

Q List two histological changes seen on biopsy in coeliac disease   2 marks

1. _____

2. _____

Q Which rash is associated with coeliac disease?   2 marks

1. _____

Q List three food groups that James will now have to avoid   3 marks

1. _____

2. _____

3. _____

Q **Give three complications of coeliac disease** 3 marks

1. _____

2. _____

3. _____

Total 20 marks

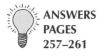

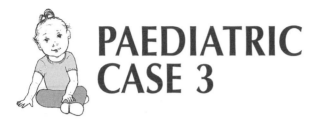

PAEDIATRIC CASE 3

Rebecca is born at 40 weeks' gestation by normal vaginal delivery weighing 3.2 kg. Her mother (gravida 1, para 1) went into labour spontaneously and labour was not prolonged. Rebecca's Apgar scores were 9 and 10 at 1 and 5 minutes, respectively, and she was transferred to the postnatal ward together with her mother. At the postnatal check the next day, the midwife notices that Rebecca's skin and sclerae are yellow. Apart from that she appears very well and is breast-feeding satisfactorily.

Q Are you concerned about Rebecca's jaundice and briefly explain your reasoning?   **2 marks**

1. _____

2. _____

Q Give three reasons why jaundice is common in neonates   **3 marks**

1. _____

2. _____

3. _____

Rebecca's jaundice is investigated. Her blood results are shown in the table.

Hb (g/dL)	12.2 (range 14.5–21.5)	Rebecca's blood group	A, Rh −ve
Platelets (× 10⁹/L)	220 (range 150–400)	Maternal blood group	O, Rh −ve
MCV (fL)	112 (range 100–135)	Total serum bilirubin (µmol/L)	140 (range 3–17) (unconjugated)
WCC (× 10⁹/L)	14 (range 10–26)	CRP (mg/L)	< 10
Film	Normal RBCs	DCT	+ (mildly +ve)

DCT, direct Coombs' test

Q **Give three causes of elevated *conjugated* bilirubin in neonates** 3 marks

1.

2.

3.

Q **What does the direct Coombs' test (DCT) detect and what does it indicate?** 2 marks

1.

2.

Q **From the blood results, what is the cause of Rebecca's jaundice?** 2 marks

1.

Q **What is your initial management?** 1 mark

1.

Q How does phototherapy work?   1 mark

1.

If unconjugated bilirubin reaches high levels (> 360 μmol/L) it can become neurotoxic.

Q What is this neurotoxicity called?   1 mark

1.

Q Give three clinical features of this   3 marks

1.

2.

3.

Q Give two long-term complications of this   2 marks

1.

2.

Fortunately for Rebecca, phototherapy is successful and she joins her new family at home 4 days later on oral folic acid. She is followed up 2 weeks later in outpatients for a repeat full blood count (FBC) to ensure that late haemolysis is not occurring.

Total   20 marks

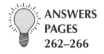

ANSWERS
PAGES
262–266

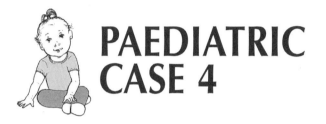

PAEDIATRIC CASE 4

Sarah is a 15-month-old, happy toddler who has just started to walk. Mum has noticed recently that when Sarah walks she seems to drag her left foot. Sarah appears unaware of this and does not complain of any pain. She was born full term with a normal vaginal delivery and there were no antenatal or postnatal problems.

Q **With regard to her motor milestones, at what ages would you expect Sarah to do the following?**   **7 marks**

1. Crawl:

2. Walk:

3. Run:

4. Kick a ball:

5. Ride a tricycle:

6. Hop on one foot:

7. Climb stairs adult fashion:

Q **Name four pathological gaits in children**   **2 marks**

1.

2.

3.

4.

Paediatrics

Q List six questions that you want to ask Mum   3 marks

1.

2.

3.

4.

5.

6.

Q What is your differential diagnosis?   2 marks

1.

2.

3.

4.

Q Which diagnosis needs immediate intervention?   1 mark

1.

Q What two manoeuvres can you do to test for congenital hip problems in neonates?   1 mark

1.

2.

Your next patient also presents with a limp – a 12-year-old boy whose weight lies on the 90th centile and who has been complaining for several weeks of an intermittent limp and knee pain, making cycling painful.

Q What is the most likely diagnosis from this history?   **1 mark**

1. _____

Q What is the typical finding on examination of the hip?   **2 marks**

1. _____

Q Which other hip pathology in a child is associated with avascular necrosis?   **1 mark**

1. _____

Total   **20 marks**

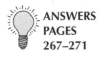
ANSWERS
PAGES
267–271

Paediatrics

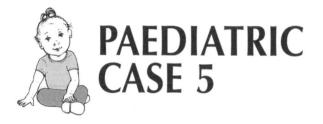

PAEDIATRIC CASE 5

Nathan is an 11-month-old infant who has been referred to the paediatric assessment unit with a history of irritability and inconsolable crying for the last 8 hours. His mother has noted that he will settle down for a few minutes but then wake up and cry loudly, drawing his legs up to his abdomen. There is no fever, vomiting or diarrhoea. His bowels were last open yesterday and his stools were normal. Past medical history is unremarkable except that Nathan is recovering from gastroenteritis and remains off his feed.

Q List five causes of inconsolable crying in an infant   5 marks

1.

2.

3.

4.

5.

Q Define infantile colic   2 marks

1.

Nathan is alert, pink and well perfused. His abdomen is not distended, and is soft with normal bowel sounds and a palpable mass in the right upper quadrant.

Q **What is intussusception?**   1 mark

1. _____

Q **In which part of the bowel does intussusception most commonly occur?**   1 mark

1. _____

Q **Name four predisposing factors for intussusception**   4 marks

1. _____

2. _____

3. _____

4. _____

Q **Name six features of intussusception**   3 marks

1. _____

2. _____

3. _____

4. _____

5. _____

6. _____

Suspecting that Nathan has intussusception, you request an abdominal ultrasound scan, shown below.

Paediatrics

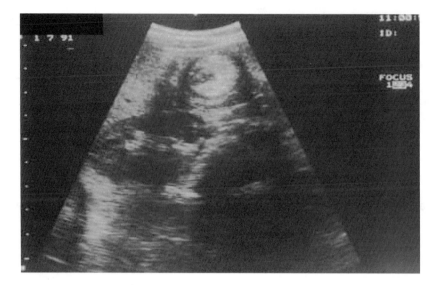

Q **What does the ultrasound show?** 2 marks

1.

Q **How would you treat intussusception in Nathan?** 2 marks

1.

Total 20 marks

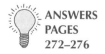

ANSWERS
PAGES
272–276

RENAL CASES:
QUESTIONS

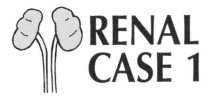 **RENAL CASE 1**

Shelia, a 49-year-old woman, is investigated for malaise and fatigue by her GP. Her current medications are insulin (for type 1 diabetes), angiotensin-converting enzyme (ACE) inhibitor (for hypertension) and non-steroidal anti-inflammatory drug (NSAID) (for chronic back pain). Her blood results are shown in the table.

Hb (g/dL)	9.2	Na^+ (mmol/L)	136
MCV (fL)	86	K^+ (mmol/L)	5.7
WCC ($\times 10^9$/L)	5.2	Urea (mmol/L)	27
Platelets ($\times 10^9$/L)	280	Creatinine (μmol/L)	245
Glucose (mmol/L)	18.7	Adjusted Ca^{2+} (mmol/L)	1.82
HbA1c (%)	9.2	PO_4^{3-} (mmol/L)	2.72

HbA1c, glycated haemoglobin; MCV, mean corpuscular volume; WCC, white cell count.

Q How much fluid is filtered through the glomerulus each day?   **1 mark**

1. _____

Q Outline four functions of the kidney   **4 marks**

1. _____

2. _____

3. _____

4. _____

Q List three blood tests suggestive of chronic renal failure (CRF) 3 marks

1.

2.

3.

Q What is the likely cause of Shelia's anaemia? 1 mark

1.

Q Name two factors that might be contributing to her renal failure 2 marks

1.

2.

Q List four *systemic* causes of pruritus 2 marks

1.

2.

3.

4.

Shelia is referred to a nephrologist for her CRF, and is kept under review for progression of her disease and to prevent or treat any complications.

Q List two treatments to prevent renal bone disease 2 marks

1.

2.

Q **How would you monitor the effectiveness of such treatment?** 1 mark

1.

A graph of Shelia's reciprocal plasma creatinine against time is shown.

RENAL FUNCTION

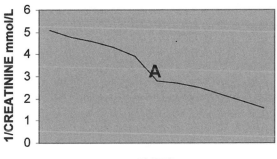

Q **Give four possible causes for the sharp decline at time A** 4 marks

1.

2.

3.

4.

Total 20 marks

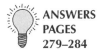 **ANSWERS
PAGES
279–284**

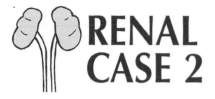

RENAL
CASE 2

Christopher, a 74-year-old man, is admitted with a 2-day history of worsening oliguria and general malaise. On examination he is hypotensive, pyrexial and clinically dehydrated. His admission urea and electrolytes (U&Es) are: Na^+ 133 mmol/L, K^+ 6.7 mmol/L, urea 41 mmol/L and creatinine 443 µmol/L. With regard to his past medical history, he is normally fit and well, taking ibuprofen for back pain and an ACE inhibitor for hypertension.

Q List two causes each of pre-renal, renal and post-renal failure   **6 marks**

Pre-renal failure:

1.

2.

Renal failure:

1.

2.

Post-renal failure:

1.

2.

Q What test can be used to distinguish between pre-renal failure and acute tubular necrosis (ATN)?   **1 mark**

1.

Christopher is diagnosed with acute renal failure (ARF) secondary to sepsis. He is resuscitated with intravenous crystalloid, started on broad-spectrum antibiotics and his nephrotoxic drugs are stopped.

Q Outline how ACE inhibitors and NSAIDs cause ARF　　　2 marks

1. ACE inhibitors:

2. NSAIDs:

Appropriate investigations are taken including an ECG, as shown.

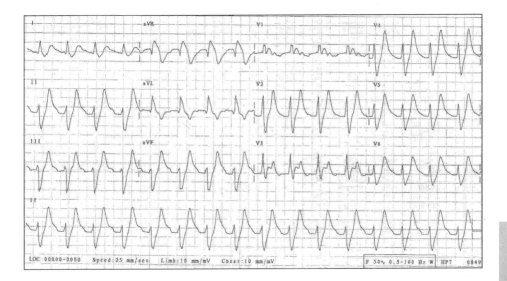

Q Give two ECG changes associated with hyperkalaemia　　　1 mark

1.

2.

Q List four causes of hyperkalaemia　　　2 marks

1.

2.

3.

4.

Q **How would you treat life-threatening hyperkalaemia?**   3 marks

1.

2.

3.

Q **List four indications for renal replacement therapy**   4 marks

1.

2.

3.

4.

Christopher's blood pressure and urine output respond to fluid resuscitation and his U&Es subsequently indicate recovery of his renal function.

Q **Name two early complications following recovery from ATN**   1 mark

1.

2.

Total   20 marks

ANSWERS
PAGES
285–290

Renal

RESPIRATORY CASES: QUESTIONS

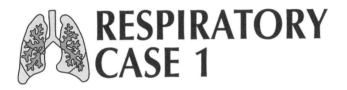 # RESPIRATORY
CASE 1

Lucy, a 21-year-old with asthma, presents to the accident and emergency department (A&E) with a 2-day history of increased shortness of breath, wheeze and cough. On examination her pulse is 125 beats/min, blood pressure 130/80 mmHg, respiratory rate 30/min, and there is widespread bilateral expiratory wheeze and reduced air entry throughout.

Q What three brief questions would you ask?   3 marks

1.

2.

3.

Q List three criteria used to indicate a severe asthma attack   3 marks

1.

2.

3.

Q List three criteria used to indicate a life-threatening asthma attack   3 marks

1.

2.

3.

Q What is your immediate management in *severe* asthma? 3 marks

1. _____

2. _____

3. _____

Q Other than in life-threatening asthma when else is intravenous magnesium sulphate used? 1 mark

1. _____

2. _____

Lucy's arterial blood gases (ABGs; on 40 per cent O_2) are shown in the table.

pH	7.38 (7.35–7.45)
Po_2 (kPa)	11.2 (> 10.6)
Pco_2 (kPa)	3.4 (4.7–6)
HCO_3^- (mmol/L)	24 (22–28)
Base excess (BE)	−1.2 (±2)

Q List two ABG markers of a *life-threatening* attack 1 mark

1. _____

2. _____

Q Give two reasons why you would request a chest radiograph 1 mark

1. _____

2. _____

Respiratory

Lucy is diagnosed with a severe asthma attack and is treated appropriately.

Q **List two ways in which the effects of treatment can be assessed non-invasively**   **1 mark**

1. _____

2. _____

Lucy's breathing improves and she is transferred to the wards.

Q **What four things should Lucy have before discharge?**   **4 marks**

1. _____

2. _____

3. _____

4. _____

Total   **20 marks**

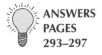

ANSWERS
PAGES
293–297

Respiratory

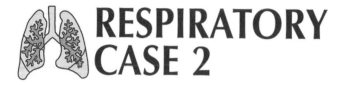

RESPIRATORY CASE 2

Tom, a 73-year-old lifelong smoker with known chronic obstructive pulmonary disease (COPD), is admitted to A&E with severe dyspnoea and cough productive of green sputum. On examination his temperature is 37°C, pulse 95 beats/min, respiratory rate 35/min, he has widespread expiratory wheeze and reduced air entry throughout, and he is cyanosed.

Q List four differential diagnoses　　　　　　　　**2 marks**

1.

2.

3.

4.

Q What four brief questions would you ask about his COPD?　　**2 marks**

1.

2.

3.

4.

Q What is your immediate management?　　　　　**3 marks**

1.

2.

3.

Q **What four non-invasive investigations would you do?**　　　　2 marks

1.

2.

3.

4.

The ABG results (on air) are shown in the table.

pH	7.37 (7.35–7.45)
Po_2 (kPa)	6.9 (> 10.6)
Pco_2 (kPa)	4.2 (4.7–6)
HCO_3^- (mmol/L)	25 (22–28)
BE	−1.2 (±2)

Q **What do the ABGs indicate?**　　　　2 marks

1.

Q **How will these results influence your immediate management?**　　　　1 mark

1.

Q **List four signs of hypercapnia**　　　　2 marks

1.

2.

3. _____

4. _____

The diagnosis is made of infective COPD exacerbation, which is successfully treated with amoxicillin.

Q What two organisms are commonly responsible for COPD exacerbations? 2 marks

1. _____

2. _____

Q On discharge, list four issues to be addressed in collaboration with Tom's GP 2 marks

1. _____

2. _____

3. _____

4. _____

Q List two qualifying criteria for home O$_2$ therapy 2 marks

1. _____

2. _____

Total 20 marks

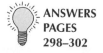

ANSWERS
PAGES
298–302

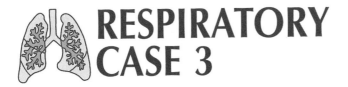# RESPIRATORY
CASE 3

*Charlotte, a 36-year-old woman, presents to A&E with sudden
onset of severe right-sided pleuritic chest pain with associated
breathlessness and feeling dizzy. She is normally fit and well, having
recently returned from a week's holiday in Florida. She is not on any
prescribed medicines except the combined oral contraceptive pill.
On examination she has a tender, swollen, right calf.*

Q List six risk factors for pulmonary embolism (PE) 3 marks

1.

2.

3.

4.

5.

6.

Q List three differential diagnoses for a tender, swollen calf 3 marks

1.

2.

3.

Q What six investigations would you do?   6 marks

1.

2.

3.

4.

5.

6.

Charlotte's ECG is shown.

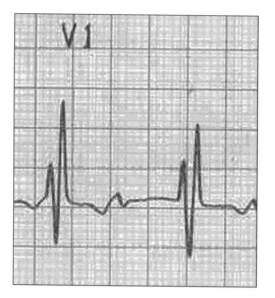

Q What does this ECG show?   2 marks

1.

The diagnosis of PE secondary to a deep vein thrombosis (DVT) is made. Charlotte is discharged on a 3-month course of warfarin with a target INR (international normalised ratio) of 2–3 and an anticoagulant card to carry.

Q **What four pieces of general advice would you give to prevent a DVT during a plane flight?**   **2 marks**

1.

2.

3.

4.

Q **What is the mechanism of action of warfarin?**   **1 mark**

1.

Six weeks later Charlotte is treated for a minor chest infection by her GP with erythromycin (an enzyme inhibitor).

Q **Is she at risk, if so of what and how should this be assessed?**   **3 marks**

1.

2.

3.

Respiratory

Total   **20 marks**

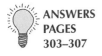

ANSWERS PAGES
303–307

111

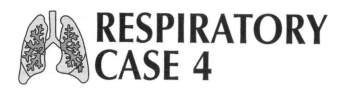# RESPIRATORY CASE 4

Margaret, a 64-year-old heavy smoker, visits her GP complaining of a 3-month history of cough associated with haemoptysis.

Q **List three respiratory causes of haemoptysis**　　　　3 marks

1.

2.

3.

Q **List two other common presenting lung cancer symptoms**　　　　2 marks

1.

2.

On examination the only abnormal finding is that she has clubbing.

Q **List two cardiac, two respiratory and two gastrointestinal (GI) causes of clubbing**　　　　3 marks

Cardiac:

1.

2.

Gastrointestinal:

1.

2.

Respiratory:

1.

2.

The GP arranges an urgent chest radiograph. The radiological report notes opacification of the right apex with destruction of the second rib consistent with bronchial carcinoma. Margaret's chest radiograph is shown here.

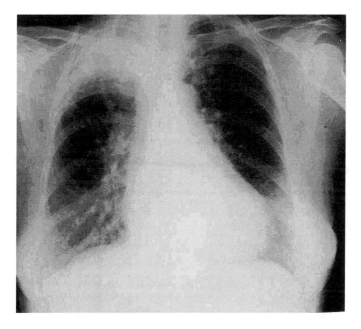

Q What is this type of lung tumour called?   1 mark

1.

Q List four signs of Horner's syndrome 2 marks

1.

2.

3.

4.

Q List four causes of round lesions of the lung on a chest radiograph 2 marks

1.

2.

3.

4.

Margaret is seen the following week as an outpatient at the respiratory clinic.

Q What two investigations would you arrange to confirm lung cancer? 2 marks

1.

2.

From these tests a diagnosis of inoperable squamous cell bronchial carcinoma is confirmed. Three months later Margaret is admitted with unremitting back pain causing night-time waking. A lateral spinal radiograph confirms secondary deposits in the thoracic vertebrae. She is treated with radiotherapy and opiate analgesia. Her bone profile results are shown in the table.

Adjusted Ca²⁺ (mmol/L)	3.7 (normal range 2.12–2.65)
PO₄³⁻ (mmol/L)	1.4 (normal range 0.8–1.45)
ALP (IU)	190 (normal range 30–150)

ALP, alkaline phosphatase.

Q List four causes of raised serum calcium   **4 marks**

1. _____

2. _____

3. _____

4. _____

Q How would you treat Margaret's hypercalcaemia?   **1 mark**

1. _____

2. _____

Total   **20 marks**

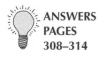

ANSWERS
PAGES
308–314

Respiratory

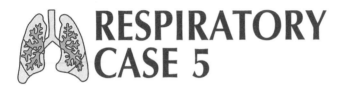

RESPIRATORY
CASE 5

John, a 72 year old insulin dependent diabetic, attends his GP with a 3-day history of cough, dyspnoea and general malaise. He is prescribed amoxicillin but continues to deteriorate and is admitted to hospital the following day. John's chest radiograph is shown here.

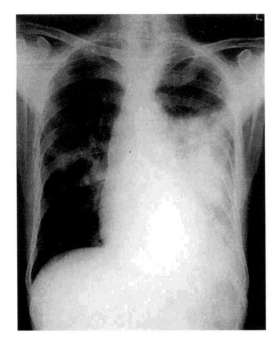

Q What is your diagnosis?   1 mark

1. _____

Q List two poor prognostic features in the history above   2 marks

1. _____

2. _____

Respiratory

A full examination is performed and appropriate investigations undertaken.

Q List three findings on *examination* that would indicate severe pneumonia   **3 marks**

1.

2.

3.

Q List three findings on *investigation* that would indicate severe pneumonia   **3 marks**

1.

2.

3.

John is diagnosed with severe pneumonia and treated with intravenous cefuroxime and clarithromycin (to cover atypical organisms).

Q List three causes of 'atypical' pneumonia   **3 marks**

1.

2.

3.

Microbiology call the ward to report Gram-positive cocci in John's blood while awaiting culture and sensitivity.

Respiratory

Q **What is the most likely cause of John's pneumonia and how can this be prevented?** 2 marks

1. _____

2. _____

Q **List six parameters used to assess treatment progress** 3 marks

1. _____

2. _____

3. _____

4. _____

5. _____

6. _____

John fails to make good progress and clinical examination reveals reduced breath sounds at the right base. His chest radiograph is repeated, which shows a right pleural effusion.

Q **What is the most likely complication?** 1 mark

1. _____

Q **How should this be treated?** 2 marks

1. _____

2. _____

Total 20 marks

ANSWERS
PAGES
315–319

Respiratory

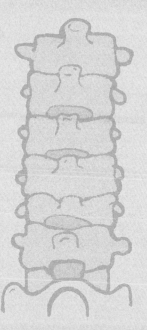

RHEUMATOLOGY
CASES: QUESTIONS

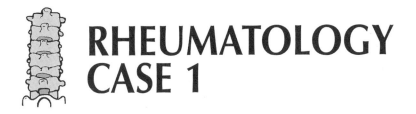

RHEUMATOLOGY CASE 1

Hayley, a 36-year-old woman, attends her GP with a 2-month history of stiff, painful, swollen hands associated with general malaise.

Q List four *inflammatory* causes of *poly*arthropathy   4 marks

1.

2.

3.

4.

Examination of Hayley's hands and wrists shows changes characteristic of rheumatoid arthritis (RA).

Q Give eight features of RA in the hands and wrists on examination   4 marks

1.

2.

3.

4.

5.

6.

7.

8.

Hayley is sent for a radiograph of her hands.

Q **Give four radiological changes in the hands in RA**　　　　2 marks

1.

2.

3.

4.

Q **List four criteria on history, examination and investigation used to diagnose RA**　　　　4 marks

1.

2.

3.

4.

Q **List four features associated with a poor prognosis**　　　　2 marks

1.

2.

3.

4.

Hayley is diagnosed with RA and started on non-steroidal anti-inflammatory drugs (NSAIDs) by her GP. She is also referred to a rheumatologist for consideration of a disease-modifying anti-rheumatic drug (DMARD).

Q **Name two DMARDs and two side effects associated with each**   **4 marks**

1.

2.

Total   **20 marks**

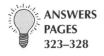
ANSWERS PAGES 323–328

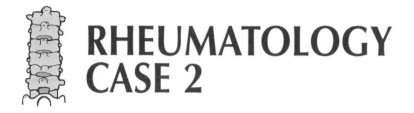

RHEUMATOLOGY CASE 2

Julie is a 28-year-old woman with a past history of depression. She attends her GP complaining of fatigue and joint pains for the last 2 months. On examination she has a butterfly facial rash.

Q How else may systemic lupus erythematosus (SLE) present?　　4 marks

1.

2.

3.

4.

Q List eight investigations that you would request　　8 marks

1.

2.

3.

4.

5.

6.

7.

8.

Julie's blood tests show a strongly positive ANA titre. She also has a raised erythrocyte sedimentation rate (ESR). Urinalysis shows 3+ proteinuria.

Q What is the likely cause of Julie's proteinuria?   1 mark

1.

Q List three treatment options for Julie's joint symptoms   3 marks

1.

2.

3.

Two years later Julie is doing well, and speaks to her GP about the possibility of becoming pregnant.

Q What are the potential problems that Julie might face during her pregnancy?   4 marks

1.

2.

3.

4.

Total   20 marks

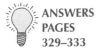

ANSWERS
PAGES
329–333

Rheumatology

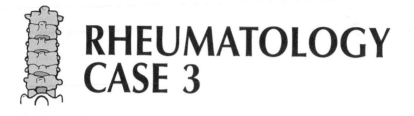

RHEUMATOLOGY CASE 3

Mabel, a 78-year-old woman, attends her GP complaining of pain and stiffness affecting her shoulder, neck and hips. She is unable to sleep at night because of the pain, and has great difficulty in getting out of bed and dressing in the mornings.

Q What blood test would confirm the probable diagnosis of polymyalgia rheumatica (PMR)? 2 marks

1. _____

Mabel's GP prescribes prednisolone 15 mg daily. However, she decides not to collect the prescription because she has fears about taking steroids. Two weeks later she represents complaining of headache, jaw ache while eating and scalp tenderness when combing her hair.

Q What would be your next steps in management? 3 marks

1. _____

2. _____

3. _____

Q What steps could have been taken to encourage Mabel to comply with her initial treatment?   4 marks

1.

2.

3.

Q Give eight complications of long-term oral steroid treatment   4 marks

1.

2.

3.

4.

5.

6.

7.

8.

Mabel agrees to start her steroid therapy, and has a rapid improvement in symptoms. She is advised that she is going to need to remain on steroid therapy for 12–18 months at least.

Q **What steps can be taken to reduce her risk of an osteoporotic fracture?**   **5 marks**

1. _____

2. _____

3. _____

4. _____

5. _____

Mabel is commenced on a once-weekly oral bisphosphonate.

Q **What is the major potential adverse effect of bisphosphonate therapy?**   **2 marks**

1. _____

Total   **20 marks**

ANSWERS
PAGES
334–337

CARDIOVASCULAR
CASES: ANSWERS

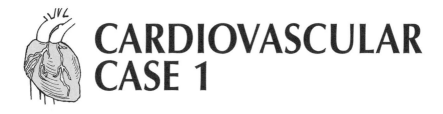

CARDIOVASCULAR CASE 1

*James, a 68-year-old lifelong smoker, is brought into A&E by
ambulance. He has a 45-minute history of central, crushing
chest pain associated with nausea, dyspnoea and sweating. On
cardiovascular examination, his blood pressure is 164/96 mmHg,
heart rate 92 beats/min and regular; JVP is 4 cm above the sternal
angle, heart sounds are normal and the chest is clear.*

Q List six differential diagnoses   **3 marks**

1. **Myocardial infarction (MI)/acute coronary syndrome (ACS – see below).**

2. **Angina pectoris.**

3. **Pulmonary embolism.**

4. **Aortic dissection.**

5. **Gastro-oesophageal reflux disease.**

6. **Pericarditis.**

7. **Musculoskeletal chest pain.**

❶ ACS encompasses unstable angina, non-ST-elevation myocardial infarction
(NSTEMI) and ST-elevation myocardial infarction (STEMI). Although similar
in their presentation their management differs. Therefore, the two key
investigations are ECG (is there any ST elevation?) and troponin (troponin
is elevated 12 hours after myocardial damage); unstable angina is not
associated with an elevated troponin, whereas an NSTEMI is.

James's ECG is shown:

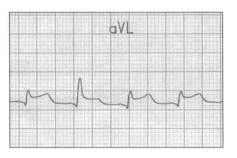

Q What is the abnormality?   1 mark

1. ST-segment elevation.

❶ Other causes of ST-segment elevation include acute pericarditis (saddle-shaped ST elevation) and left ventricular aneurysm (ST elevation in leads V1–6).

❶ Other investigations include chest radiograph (to exclude pulmonary causes of chest pain; signs of LVF) and bloods (full blood count [FBC], urea and electrolytes [U&Es], glucose, lipids).

This abnormality is seen in leads I, aVL and V5–6.

Q What is the most likely diagnosis?   2 marks

1. Lateral wall MI.

❶ The leads affected reflect the site of the infarct: inferior (II, III, aVF), anterior (V1–4), posterior (ST depression in V1–3 with dominant R waves). New-onset left bundle-branch block (LBBB) is usually the result of a large anterior infarct.

Q What other ECG changes may be expected to develop?   1 mark

1. T-wave inversion (within 24 hours).

2. Pathological Q waves (within days): pathological Q waves do not appear with subendocardial (not extending through the ventricular wall) MIs.

❶ ST elevation rarely persists unless a left ventricular aneurysm develops.

❶ ECG changes present in other forms of ACS include ST depression, T-wave flattening or inversion, non-specific changes or normal ECG.

Q What is your immediate management? 3 marks

1. **Intravenous diamorphine (+ antiemetic): provides analgesia plus vasodilatation.**

2. **O_2: to ensure maximal oxygenation of the myocardium.**

3. **Sublingual glyceryl trinitrate or GTN (spray or tablets): to ensure maximal coronary artery vasodilatation.**

4. **Aspirin (300 mg chewed if not given already) or clopidogrel if aspirin is contraindicated: aspirin and clopidogrel both prevent platelet aggregation via inhibition of thromboxane A_2 formation and the ADP receptor, respectively.**

5. **Intravenous β blocker (unless contraindicated, e.g. bradycardia, uncontrolled heart failure, asthma): reduces risk of LV rupture in the first week.**

6. **Thrombolysis, e.g. with tenecteplase (TNK): to achieve reperfusion of coronary arteries. Ideally 'door-to-needle time' should be < 30 minutes.**

❶ The acronym MONA refers to morphine, oxygen, nitrates and aspirin.

❶ It is important to appreciate that the effects of antiplatelet agents and thrombolysis are additive, and that all patients should receive antiplatelets irrespective of whether thrombolysis is given.

❶ Primary angioplasty is at least as effective as thrombolysis and is offered in some hospitals. While waiting for PCI (percutaneous coronary intervention) give a GPIIb/IIIa receptor inhibitor infusion, which prevents platelet aggregation.

❶ The management of ACS without ST elevation differs from STEMI in that thrombolysis is not indicated. Instead patients are anticoagulated with low-molecular-weight heparins (LMWH).

The patient undergoes thrombolysis within 4 hours.

Q List two ECG indications for thrombolysis   2 marks

1. ST-segment elevation > 2 mm in two contiguous chest leads.

2. ST-segment elevation > 1 mm in two limb leads.

3. New-onset LBBB.

4. True posterior infarct (ST depression V1–3 with elevation > 1 mm in posterior leads V7–9).

❶ Thrombolysis is effective only if given within 12 hours of onset of chest pain or if is there ongoing chest pain. Consider re-thrombolysis or rescue angioplasty if thrombolysis fails to reperfuse within 60–90 minutes as demonstrated by < 50 per cent resolution of ST elevation.

Q Name three absolute contraindications for thrombolysis   3 marks

1. Previous haemorrhagic cerebrovascular accident (CVA).

2. Recent CVA within last 6 months.

3. Intracranial neoplasm.

4. Recent serious trauma, head injury or surgery (within 3 weeks).

5. Active bleeding (not menstrual).

6. Suspected aortic dissection: widened mediastinum on chest radiograph, unequal arm BP.

7. Uncontrolled severe hypertension, e.g. > 200/120 mmHg.

Q List five complications of myocardial infarction   5 marks

1. Cardiac arrest.

2. LVF: usually the result of an anterior MI.

3. Right ventricular failure (RVF): usually the result of an inferior MI. Causes hypotension; treatment is fluids.

4. Arrhythmias/heart block, e.g. ventricular tachycardias (VTs; common during reperfusion), atrial fibrillation (AF), bradyarrhythmias (may require atropine

or temporary transcutaneous/intravenous pacemaker if symptomatic). Hence all ACS patients should ideally be managed on coronary care with cardiac monitoring.

5. Systemic embolism: may arise from a LV mural thrombus.

6. LV aneurysm formation.

7. Mitral regurgitation, e.g. caused by papillary muscle rupture.

8. Pericarditis (Dressler's syndrome).

9. Ventricular septal defect (VSD).

James is discharged 5 days later with no complications.

Q What advice, treatment and investigations would you recommend to reduce his risk of a similar episode?   5 marks

1. Echocardiogram: to assess any structural/functional heart defects.

2. Exercise ECG: post-MI risk stratification, i.e. a positive test indicates residual ischaemia.

3. Coronary angiogram (if exercise test is positive) ± angioplasty/stenting.

4. Address any modifiable risk factors, e.g. smoking, diabetes, hypertension.

5. Supervised cardiac rehabilitation.

6. ACE inhibitor: minimises LV impairment.

7. Aspirin (75 mg daily): reduces risk of all vascular events (+ clopidogrel – continue clopidogrel for 5 days for STEMI and 12 months for NSTEMI).

8. β Blocker: reduces mortality in patients with MI. If contraindicated consider a calcium channel blocker.

9. Statin therapy: shown to improve prognosis regardless of baseline cholesterol levels.

Total   25 marks

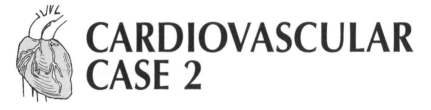

CARDIOVASCULAR CASE 2

Sarah, a 77-year-old woman, attends A&E complaining of palpitations. Her ECG is shown below.

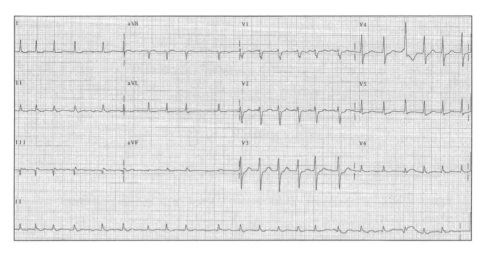

Q What does the ECG show?   2 marks

1. Atrial fibrillation.

ⓘ AF is diagnosed by absent P waves and irregular QRS complexes. AF results from a chaotic irregular atrial rhythm (300–600 beats/min) of which only a proportion are sufficient to generate an action potential that is conducted to the ventricles, causing an irregular ventricular rate.

ⓘ AF may present with symptoms of palpitations, breathlessness and chest pain. However, the majority of presentations are clinically silent with the first presentation as a CVA, heart failure or incidental ECG finding.

Q List six causes of this rhythm   3 marks

1. Hypertension.

2. Ischaemic heart disease.

? QUESTIONS PAGES 6–8

3. Myocardial infarction.

4. Hyperthyroidism.

5. Valvular heart disease (particularly mitral valve disease).

6. Pneumonia.

7. Pulmonary embolism.

8. Alcohol excess.

9. Heart failure.

10. Lone atrial fibrillation, i.e. no identifiable cause.

11. Cardiomyopathy.

Q What six other investigations would you do?   3 marks

1. U&Es: any electrolyte imbalance, e.g. hypokalaemia may cause arrhythmia.

2. Thyroid function tests: to exclude hyperthyroidism.

3. Chest radiograph: to exclude heart failure, pneumonia.

4. Troponin: to exclude MI.

5. Echocardiogram: e.g. to assess valvular disease, identify underlying cardiomyopathy, assess LV function.

6. 24-hour ECG: is AF persistent or paroxysmal (see below)?

❶ AF can be classified as acute, *paroxysmal* (episodes of AF that terminate spontaneously), *persistent* (terminated either pharmacologically or electrically – see below) or *permanent* (fails to respond to attempts to cardiovert or when cardioversion is deemed inappropriate).

Q What two drugs may be used for rate control?   2 marks

1. β Blockers, e.g. atenolol.

2. (Rate-limiting) calcium channel blocker (diltiazem or verapamil).

3. Digoxin.

❶ The treatment of AF involves either *rhythm* or *rate* control. First-line treatment in *paroxysmal* AF is rhythm control; in *permanent* AF it is rate control. The decision whether to rate or rhythm control in *persistent* AF depends on age, whether AF is symptomatic, existing IHD, evidence of heart failure (cardioversion improves LV function) and suitability for cardioversion (e.g. contraindications to anticoagulation).

❶ If patients are rate controlled, first-line treatment is either a standard β blocker or a calcium channel blocker. Digoxin should be considered as monotherapy only in predominantly sedentary patients (it is ineffective in controlling AF during exertion). Amiodarone is not recommended for rate control in AF (although it can be used for rate control in an acute setting).

Q What two methods may be used to attempt cardioversion 2 marks

1. Chemical cardioversion, i.e. with anti-arrhythmic drugs.

2. DC cardioversion.

❶ In acute AF (< 48 hours) use either chemical or DC cardioversion; in more established AF, DC cardioversion is first-line treatment.

❶ If AF is acute there is no need to anticoagulate before chemical or DC cardioconversion; otherwise anticoagulate 3 weeks before and 4 weeks after cardioconversion (clearly this does not apply to haemodynamically compromised patients who require urgent DC cardioversion). If the patient is at high risk of attempted DC cardioversion being unsuccessful (e.g. previous failure), pre-treatment with anti-arrhythmic drugs before DC cardioversion increases the likelihood of restoring and maintaining sinus rhythm. Intravenous amiodarone is first-line in those with structural heart disease and flecainide in those without.

Q What two drugs may be used for rhythm control? 2 marks

1. Standard β blockers.

2. Class 1 anti-arrhythmic, i.e. flecainide, propafenone.

3. Class 3 anti-arrhythmic, i.e. sotalol, amiodarone.

❶ Several anti-arrhythmic drugs can be used to maintain sinus rhythm in patients with paroxysmal or persistent AF who have been successfully cardioverted. First-line treatment is a standard β blocker; class 1 or 3 anti-arrhythmics are reserved in treatment failures.

❶ Digoxin is not indicated for rhythm control and may actually be pro-arrhythmic.

Q What class of anti-arrhythmic is amiodarone in?　　　　　　　2 marks

1. Class 3 anti-arrhythmic.

❶ Anti-arrhythmic drugs are classified according to the changes they cause in the action potential.

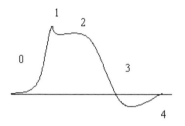

❶ 0 – rapid depolarisation caused by opening of fast Na^+ channels
1 – early repolarisation caused by closure of Na^+ channels and opening of K^+ channels
2 – plateau phase where K^+ outflux equals Ca^{2+} influx as a result of opening of slow Ca^{2+} channels
3 – late repolarisation after closure of Ca^{2+} channels
4 – return to resting membrane potential by Na^+/K^+ ATPtase
Class 1 (further divided into 1a, 1b, 1c): slow phase 0, e.g. flecainide (1c)
Class 2: slow phase 4, i.e. standard β blockers
Class 3: slow phase 3, e.g. amiodarone, sotalol
Class 4: calcium channel blockers; more effective in supraventricular tachycardia (SVT) where the action potential in the atrioventricular (AV) (and sinoatrial [SA]) node is generated by Ca^{2+} influx as opposed to Na^+ influx in the myocardium.

Q List three side effects of amiodarone　　　　　　　3 marks

1. **Hypothyroidism: reduces the peripheral conversion of thyroxine (T_4) to triiodothyronine (T_3).**

2. **Hyperthyroidism.**

3. **Pro-arrhythmic: lengthens the Q–T interval.**

4. **Pulmonary fibrosis.**

5. **Peripheral neuropathy.**

6. **Hepatitis.**

7. **Greyish skin pigmentation.**

8. **Skin photosensitivity.**

9. **Corneal deposits.**

❶ Amiodarone has a very long half-life (approximately 50 days) and so, if prescribed orally, it takes weeks to have its effect. When initiating therapy a loading dose is given: 200 mg three times daily for 1 week, 200 mg twice daily for 1 week, then maintenance therapy of 200 mg once daily. If a rapid effect is required, it is given by intravenous infusion (ideally by central line as irritant to veins): 300 mg over 1 hour, then 900 mg over 24 hours.

Q **Name three complications if her rhythm is not appropriately treated** 3 marks

1. **CVA (stroke).**

2. **Heart failure.**

3. **Syncope.**

4. **Angina.**

❶ The main risk is embolic stroke. Age, heart failure, vascular disease (IHD, peripheral vascular disease or PVD), diabetes, hypertension and previous transient ischaemic attack (TIA)/CVA all increase the risk.

Q **What drug is used for anticoagulation, how is it monitored and what is the target range?** 3 marks

1. **Warfarin.**

2. **INR (international normalised ratio – normal range 0.9–1.2); calculated by comparing the prothrombin time (PT) of the patient with a standard value.**

3. **2–3.**

❶ The decision whether to anticoagulate a patient in paroxysmal, persistent or permanent AF depends on their risk of stroke, assessed on the basis of the risk factors above. AF carries a risk of embolic stroke of 2–4 per cent per year. Warfarin therapy can reduce this by around 60 per cent, compared with 30 per cent reduction with aspirin alone. Those at high risk should ideally be anticoagulated with warfarin; those at low risk can simply be treated with aspirin (75–300 mg).

Total   **25 marks**

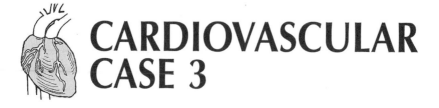

CARDIOVASCULAR CASE 3

David, a 51-year-old man, has attended his GP for his third blood pressure measurement; his three readings are 167/96, 162/104 and 174/104 mmHg.

Q **Define the systolic/diastolic ranges for mild (phase 1), moderate (phase 2) and severe (phase 3) hypertension** 3 marks

1. **Mild: 140–159/90–99.**

2. **Moderate: 160–199/100–109.**

3. **Severe: ≥ 200/110.**

❶ Treat moderate-to-severe hypertension; treat mild hypertension if target organ damage (e.g. left ventricular hypertrophy (LVH) on ECG, retinopathy), existing cardiovascular disease (CVD) or 10-year CVD risk ≥ 20 per cent (calculated on the basis of sex, smoking status and TC:HDL [total cholesterol:high-density lipoprotein] ratio – see coloured charts at the back of the *British National Formulary* or BNF).

You request an ECG, shown below:

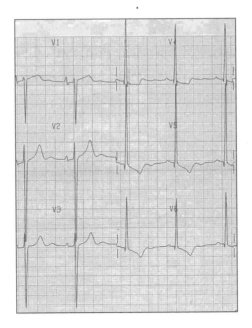

Q What does his ECG show? 1 mark

1. LVH.

❶ LVH causes tall R waves in V5–6 and deep S waves in V1–2 (consider LVH if R wave in V5–6 > 25 mm or combined R wave in V6 and S wave in V1 > 35 mm). May also get T-wave inversion in the lateral leads (i.e. I, AvL, V5–6) and left axis deviation (i.e. positive in I, negative in II and III).

Q Why is this important with regard to hypertension? 1 mark

1. LVH indicates hypertensive end-organ damage and is an indication for antihypertensive treatment even in patients with mild hypertension.

❶ In the presence of LVH request an echocardiogram to assess LV size (and function).

Q List four additional initial investigations that you would do 4 marks

1. U&Es: renal impairment (either secondary to hypertension or underlying renal disease causing hypertension), hypokalaemia may indicate Conn's syndrome.

2. **Fasting lipids: hypercholesterolaemia is an independent risk factor for CVD.**

3. **Fasting glucose: diabetes is an independent risk factor for CVD.**

4. **Urine dipstick for protein and blood: may indicate underlying renal disease (if positive send for microscopy and request KUB ultrasound scan).**

❶ Examination should include fundoscopy to assess duration and/or severity of hypertension:

Grade	Hypertensive retinopathy
I	Tortuous retinal arteries with thick shiny walls (silver wiring)
II	Arteriovenous or AV nipping (narrowing where arteries cross veins)
III	Flame haemorrhages and cotton-wool spots (small infarcts)
IV	Papilloedema

Q **List three causes of secondary hypertension**   3 marks

1. **Renal or renovascular disease, e.g. renal artery stenosis or glomerulonephritis.**

2. **Endocrine disorders: Cushing's syndrome (corticosteroid excess), Conn's syndrome (hyperaldosteronism), phaeochromocytoma (norepinephrine and epinephrine excess), acromegaly (human growth hormone [hGH] excess).**

3. **Drugs: combined oral contraceptive (COC), corticosteroids, alcohol, nonsteroidal anti-inflammatory drugs (NSAIDs).**

4. **Coarctation of the aorta.**

5. **Pregnancy.**

Q **List three reasons when you would consider referring a hypertensive patient for specialist care**   3 marks

1. **Suspicion of secondary hypertension.**

2. **Young, e.g. < 35 years old.**

3. **Impaired renal function.**

4. **Proteinuria and/or haematuria.**

5. Hypokalaemia (in the absence of diuretics).

6. Refractory hypertension to multi-medications (exclude poor compliance).

7. Accelerated phase (malignant) hypertension.

❶ Malignant hypertension refers to severe hypertension, i.e. BP > 200/120 mmHg, in the presence of grade 3 (± grade 4) hypertensive retinopathy. It often causes headache and visual disturbances. It may also cause acute renal failure, heart failure and encephalopathy, which are hypertensive emergencies. Most patients can be managed on oral therapy. Urgent lowering of BP (over days not hours) is indicated only in encephalopathy; typically use intravenous labetalol. Never use sublingual nifedipine because it can cause an uncontrolled drop in BP, causing stroke.

You determine that David's blood pressure needs to be treated.

Q What three lifestyle changes would you recommend?　　　3 marks

1. Lose weight: aim for body mass index (BMI) 20–25.

2. Stop smoking.

3. Encourage regular exercise.

4. Reduce salt consumption.

5. Reduce alcohol consumption to < 21 units/week.

6. Consume five portions of fruit and vegetables/day.

7. Reduce consumption of total and saturated fat.

Q What are the first-line antihypertensives?　　　3 marks

1. ACE inhibitor, e.g. ramipril or if unable to tolerate (ACE inhibitor can cause a chronic cough) consider an angiotension II receptor antagonist (ARA), e.g. irbesartan.

2. Ca^{2+} channel blocker, e.g. amlodipine.

3. Thiazide diuretic, e.g. bendroflumethiazide.

❶ The National Institute for Health and Clinical Excellence (NICE) guidelines recommend that, in hypertensive patients aged ≥ 55 years (or black patients of any age), first-line treatment is either a calcium channel blocker (C) or a thiazide diuretic (D); in hypertensive patients aged < 55 years first-line treatment is an ACE inhibitor (A) (black patients have low renin hypertension and thus ACE inhibitors are ineffective).

❶ β Blockers (B) used to be first-line treatment of hypertension but have been shown to be less effective (than A, C or D) at reducing major cardiovascular events, particularly stroke, and are now used in second-line treatment (see flow chart). They are also a risk factor for diabetes.

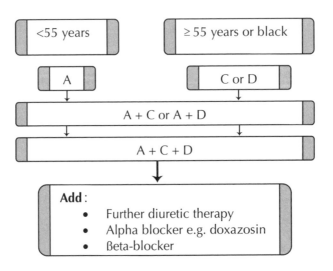

You prescribe David an ACE inhibitor.

Q What two electrolyte abnormalities may ACE inhibitors cause?   2 marks

1. **Hyperkalaemia: as a result of inhibition of aldosterone-mediated K⁺ excretion.**

2. **Raised urea and creatinine: may cause impaired renal function due to reduced renal perfusion in patients with renovascular disease; use with caution if generalised atherosclerosis or peripheral vascular disease.**

❶ When prescribing an ACE inhibitor, U&Es must be monitored at baseline, 1–2 weeks after initiation of treatment, after every increase in dose and at annual review.

❶ The renin–angiotensin system plays a major role in controlling blood pressure. The kidney secretes renin, which converts circulating angiotensin (synthesised by the liver) to angiotensin I; this, in turn is converted to angiotensin II by ACE (in the pulmonary vasculature). Angiotensin II increases blood pressure by increasing aldosterone and antidiuretic hormone (ADH) secretion, causing vasoconstriction (angiotensin II is one of the most potent endogenous vasoconstrictors) and stimulating the hypothalamic thirst centre.

Q **Name four complications if David's hypertension is not treated**　　2 marks

1. **Stroke: people with hypertension have a sixfold increased risk of stroke over people with normotension.**

2. **CVD: people with hypertension have a threefold increased risk of CVD over people with normotension.**

3. **Heart failure.**

4. **PVD (peripheral vascular disease).**

5. **Chronic renal failure: hypertensive nephropathy.**

6. **Impaired vision: hypertensive retinopathy.**

Total　　　　　　　　　　　　　　　　　　　　　　　**25 marks**

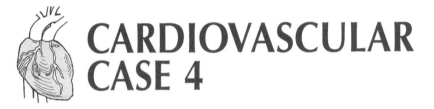

CARDIOVASCULAR CASE 4

Tim, a 60-year-old man, visits his GP complaining of recent episodes of central chest tightness on exertion. These settle on rest and last no longer than 5–10 minutes. There is nothing of note in his past medical history. Cardiovascular examination is normal.

Q The clinical suspicion is of angina pectoris. What are the main risk factors for ischaemic heart disease (IHD)?   **5 marks**

1. **Smoking.**

2. **Diet high in fat and low in fruit and vegetables.**

3. **Sedentary lifestyle.**

4. **Diabetes mellitus.**

5. **Hypertension.**

6. **Hyperlipidaemia.**

7. **Family history of IHD.**

❶ Initial investigations include:

- FBC: exclude anaemia as a cause of his angina.

- TFTs (thyroid function tests): exclude hyperthyroidism as a cause of his angina. Hypothyroidism is also an important cause of muscular chest pain.

- Glucose: to look for diabetes

- Fasting lipids: hyperlipidaemia is a risk factor for IHD.

❶ Resting ECG is of limited value in patients with stable angina and is normal in 50 per cent of patients. A chest radiograph is also unhelpful (although may reveal non-cardiac causes of chest pain or any complications of IHD, e.g. pulmonary oedema).

All of Tim's blood tests are normal except a fasting TC of 7.2 mmol/L.

Q **What is the recommended upper limit for fasting TC in the secondary prevention of IHD?** 2 marks

1. **5 mmol/L.**

❶ Patients with existing IHD should ideally have a fasting TC of ≤ 5 mmol/L (or a 30 per cent reduction, whichever is greatest) (and an LDL [low-density lipoprotein] ≤ 3 mmol/L).

Tim is prescribed a statin by his GP.

Q **What blood test must you request before prescribing a statin and what advice must you give to patients on statin therapy?** 4 marks

1. **Liver function tests (LFTs).**

❶ Statins are potentially hepatotoxic and are contraindicated in liver impairment. LFTs should be carried out at baseline and at regular intervals thereafter; treatment should be discontinued if AST/ALT (aspartate transaminase/alanine transaminase) rises to three times the upper limit (normal range is 3–35 IU/L).

2. **Patients should report any unexplained muscle pain.**

❶ Statins rarely cause myositis (diagnosed by raised creatine kinase [CK] causing muscle pain, weakness and tenderness. In severe cases this can lead to rhabdomyolysis and acute renal failure.

Tim's resting ECG is normal. His GP arranges an appointment as an outpatient for an ETT to perform a risk assessment.

Q **Indicate whether each of the following exercise ECGs represents a negative or a positive ETT** 3 marks

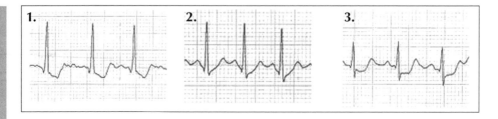

1. **ECG 1: downsloping ST depression is a positive exercise test.**

2. **EGG 2: upsloping ST depression is a negative exercise test**

3. **ECG 3: planar ST depression is a positive exercise test.**

ⓘ Most patients with a clinical diagnosis of angina will require some form of stress testing. If an ETT is inappropriate, e.g. poor mobility, stress echocardiography or myocardial perfusion scans at rest and stress (e.g. using adenosine) can identify areas of ischaemia.

ⓘ On ETT horizontal or downsloping ST depression indicates myocardial ischaemia; upsloping ST depression is a non-specific finding. Other indicators of ischaemia include chest pain, a fall in blood pressure (normally increases with exercise) and development of AV block or LBBB.

Tim's exercise tolerance test is strongly positive. His cardiologist prescribes 75 mg aspirin once daily, addresses his modifiable risk factors and places him on the waiting list for coronary angiography.

Q List four drugs that may be prescribed to control angina   4 marks

1. **Nitrates: these are vasodilators. For symptoms use sublingual GTN spray; as a prophylaxis give regular oral nitrate, e.g. isosorbide mononitrate (if given twice daily, doses need to be timed to ensure nitrate-free period to prevent tolerance).**

2. **β Blockers, e.g. atenolol: reduce heart rate (negative chronotropic effect) and force of contraction (negative inotropic effect), thereby reducing myocardial O_2 demand.**

3. **Ca^{2+} channel antagonists, e.g. amlodipine: act as both vasodilators and**

negative inotropes (thereby reducing myocardial O$_2$ demand).

4. K$^+$ channel activators, e.g. nicorandil: cause vasodilatation.

❶ In the absence of a β blocker (and normal LV function), consider a rate-limiting Ca^{2+} channel antagonist (i.e. diltiazem, verapamil) which additionally reduces heart rate; however, it should not be combined with a β blocker because they may cause heart block.

Three months later Tim undergoes angiography, which shows severe stenosis of one of his coronary arteries.

Q **What two procedures are available to treat the stenosed artery?**   2 marks

1. **Percutaneous transluminal coronary angioplasty (PTCA) ± stenting: balloon dilatation of the stenosed vessel plus insertion of a stent. Improves symptoms but not prognosis.**

2. **Coronary artery bypass grafting (CABG), e.g. using left internal mammary artery: improves symptoms and prognosis (however, it carries more complications than PTCA, e.g. perioperative MI).**

❶ Referral for coronary angiography to assess any stenosis of the coronary vessels is indicated in patients with angina refractory to medical treatment, a strongly positive ETT, unstable angina or angina post-MI.

❶ PTCA + stenting is not appropriate for certain patterns of IHD, including three-vessel disease with left anterior descending (LAD) involvement and left main stem stenosis, for which CABG is indicated.

Total   **20 marks**

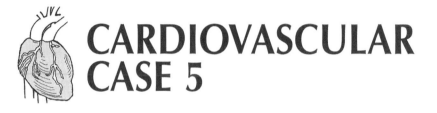

CARDIOVASCULAR CASE 5

John, a 72-year-old man, is referred by his GP to cardiac outpatients complaining of a 3-month history of progressive breathlessness. He is now breathless even when doing simple tasks around the home such as dressing. He is currently prescribed medications for his hypertension and inflammatory arthritis.

Q List four non-cardiac causes of gradually progressive dyspnoea   **2 marks**

1. **Chronic obstructive pulmonary disease (COPD).**

2. **Fibrotic lung disease, e.g. occupational lung disease, granulomatous disease, e.g. sarcoidosis, or connective tissue disease, e.g. rheumatoid arthritis.**

3. **Lung cancer.**

4. **Pleural effusion.**

5. **Anaemia.**

6. **Multiple pulmonary emboli.**

Q From the history above classify his heart failure according to the NYHA criteria   **2 marks**

1. **Grade III heart failure i.e. dyspnoea on minimal exertion.**

❶ NYHA heart failure classification

Grade	Extent of breathlessness
I	No undue breathlessness
II	Breathlessness on moderate exertion
III	Dyspnoea on minimal exertion
IV	Dyspnoea at rest; all activity causes discomfort

QUESTIONS PAGES 15–17

Q **List four symptoms suggestive of LVF** 2 marks

1. **Fatigue.**

2. **Exertional dyspnoea.**

3. **Orthopnoea: enquire about the number of pillows slept on at night.**

4. **Paroxysmal nocturnal dyspnoea (PND): patient complains of waking up with sensation of drowning.**

5. **Nocturnal cough (may bring up pink froth).**

6. **'Cardiac' wheeze.**

7. **Weight loss ('cardiac cachexia').**

❶ Heart failure can be classified as LVF or right ventricular failure (RVF); when occurring together it is termed congestive heart failure (CCF).

❶ Symptoms of RVF include fatigue, peripheral oedema, anorexia and nausea (caused by bowel oedema), abdominal distension (resulting from ascites), right upper quadrant (RUQ) pain (caused by liver congestion) and wasting (often with fluid-derived weight gain).

Q **What hormone is significantly raised in heart failure?** 1 mark

1. **B-type (or brain) natriuretic peptide (BNP).**

❶ BNP is secreted by the ventricle myocardium in response to distension and acts to reduce circulating volume by inhibiting renin, ADH and aldosterone secretion (similar actions to atrial natriuretic peptide [ANP]). Levels are significantly increased in heart failure. BNP measurement has been the subject of much research in recent years, and is shortly going to be introduced as a blood screening test for heart failure.

Q **What key investigation would you do to confirm heart failure?** 2 marks

1. **Echocardiogram: this is a key investigation in heart failure. It will confirm the diagnosis and its severity, and may indicate the cause.**

❶ Parameters assessed by echocardiography include LV function (e.g. LV ejection fraction), RV function, regional/localised hypokinesis (as a result of underlying IHD) and valvular function.

153

ⓘ Other investigations in heart failure include:

- FBC: anaemia can cause heart failure; also heart failure may cause anaemia of chronic disease (a poor prognostic marker).

- U&Es: heart failure is associated with renal impairment and electrolyte disturbances; (dilutional) hyponatraemia is a poor prognostic marker.

- Thyroid function tests (TFTs): exclude hyper-/hypothyroidism.

- LFTs: elevated in hepatic congestion.

- Ferritin: haemochromatosis is an uncommon but reversible cause of heart failure.

- Glucose and lipids: risk factors for IHD – main cause of heart failure.

- ECG: rarely normal in heart failure, e.g. Q waves (previous MI), LVH (caused by hypertension)

- Chest radiograph: cardiomegaly (cardiothoracic ratio > 0.5); exclude pulmonary causes of breathlessness

- Troponin (in an acute setting).

John is diagnosed with congestive cardiac failure. John's PA chest radiograph is shown

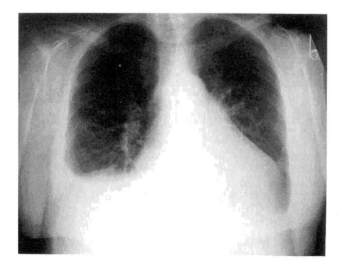

Q List two features seen on the chest radiograph 2 marks

1. **Cardiomegaly:cardiothoracic ratio > 0.5 (not possible to assess on anteroposterior or AP film).**

2. **Pleural effusions: blunting of costophrenic angles.**

3. **Upper lobe diversion: prominent vascular markings in upper lung fields as a result of redistribution of blood**

❶ There is no evidence of frank pulmonary oedema or fluid in the horizontal fissure (seen as a horizontal white line in the right lung field). Pulmonary oedema encompasses interstitial oedema, which is seen as small faint horizontal white lines at the peripheries of the lung fields (Kerley B lines), and alveolar oedema, which appears on the chest radiograph as perihilar shadowing (bats' wings).

Q List four causes of LVF 4 marks

1. **IHD: most common cause of heart failure.**

2. **Hypertension.**

3. **Left-sided valve disease, e.g. aortic stenosis, severe mitral regurgitation.**

4. **Cardiomyopathies, e.g dilated cardiomyopthy.**

❶ The main causes of RVF are secondary to LVF, cor pulmonale, pulmonary embolism (PE), right-sided valve disease and left-to-right shunts, e.g. ventricular septal defects.

John is being treated for both hypertension and inflammatory arthritis with the following medications: aspirin, verapamil, carvedilol, methotrexate and diclofenac.

Q Which of these drugs should be avoided now that a diagnosis of heart failure has been made? 2 marks

1. **Diclofenac (NSAID): promotes fluid retention by inhibiting prostaglandin-mediated Na⁺ excretion.**

2. **Verapamil: Ca²⁺ channel antagonists have a negative inotropic effect and will further suppress LV function.**

ⓘ Conversely, β blockers (e.g. bisoprolol, carvedilol), which are also negative inotropes, are introduced in *stable* heart failure in low dose with slow, stepwise titration to improve long-term prognosis.

John's cardiologist commences him on an ACE inhibitor and furosemide.

Q **List three electrolyte abnormalities caused by furosemide**   3 marks

ⓘ Furosemide is a loop diuretic that acts by inhibiting the $Na^+/K^+/Cl^-$ pump in the loop of Henle. It may cause:

1. **Hyponatraemia.**

2. **Hypocalcaemia: unlike thiazides, which are Ca²⁺-sparing diuretics.**

3. **Hypokalaemia: consider giving in combination with K⁺-sparing diuretic if problematic, although ACE inhibitors cause hyperkalaemia so not usually necessary.**

4. **Hypomagnesaemia.**

5. **Hyperuricaemia: may precipitate gout.**

ⓘ First-line treatment in heart failure is ACE inhibitors, which reduce both morbidity and mortality, followed by β blockers, then spironolactone.

ⓘ Diuretics improve symptoms in heart failure as a result of peripheral or pulmonary oedema but *do not* reduce mortality. Intravenous furosemide is used in acute pulmonary oedema to induce an immediate vasodilatation, which reduces preload and a delayed diuretic response.

ⓘ Digoxin is used for symptom control in heart failure for its positive inotropic effect (first line in AF). It acts by inhibiting the Na^+/K^+ pump (and so may cause hyponatraemia and hyperkalaemia), resulting in raised intracellular Ca^{2+} (in exchange for Na^+); this increases the force of myocardial contraction (it also stimulates parasympathetic innervation, reducing the heart rate). Digoxin has a very narrow therapeutic range; toxicity causes gastrointestinal disturbance, visual disturbance (xanthopsia

– a yellow tinge to objects) and arrhythmias, e.g. VT. This is treated by stopping digoxin, correcting any hypokalaemia and treating any arrhythmia; in life-threatening toxicity anti-digoxin antibodies (Digibind) may be used. Digoxin may cause sagging ST depression (reverse tick) although this does not necessarily indicate toxicity.

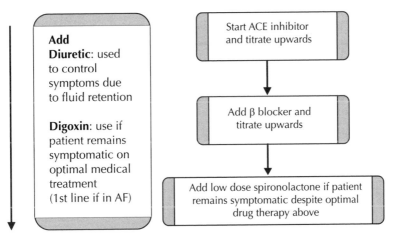

Total   **20 marks**

ENDOCRINOLOGY
CASES: ANSWERS

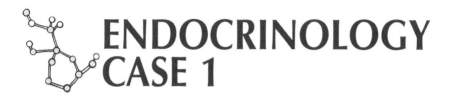

ENDOCRINOLOGY CASE 1

Gloria, a 38-year-old woman, is referred by her GP to an endocrinologist with symptoms of thyrotoxicosis.

Q **Name six symptoms that Gloria may be complaining of** 3 marks

1. **Weight loss (despite increased appetite).**

2. **Increased appetite.**

3. **Heat intolerance.**

4. **Sweating.**

5. **Fatigue and weakness.**

6. **Irritability, nervousness, restlessness, insomnia.**

7. **Diarrhoea.**

8. **Palpitations, dyspnoea, angina.**

9. **Oligomenorrhoea, loss of libido, infertility.**

❶ The thyroid gland, stimulated by TSH from the anterior pituitary, produces and releases T_4 and T_3, which exert negative feedback on TSH. The thyroid produces more T_4 than T_3, which is more biologically active; most T_4 undergoes peripheral conversion to T_3. Thyroid hormones are over 95 per cent protein bound, predominantly to thyroxine-binding globulin (TBG), although it is the unbound (i.e. free) form that is biologically active. Thyroid hormones regulate cell metabolism, enhance the effects of catecholamines, and regulate growth and mental development.

❶ Thyrotoxicosis is the result of excessive levels of circulating free thyroxine (FT_4) and/or free triiodothyronine (FT_3). Hyperthyroidism refers to an overactive thyroid gland although thyrotoxicosis can occur without hyperthyroidism, e.g. excessive thyroxine administration.

**QUESTIONS
PAGES
21–23**

On examination she is in sinus tachycardia, and has a fine tremor and bulging eyes (exophthalmos).

Q List four signs specific to Graves' disease 2 marks

ⓘ Signs of thyrotoxicosis include sinus tachycardia, atrial fibrillation (particularly in older patients), warm moist peripheries, fine tremor, lid lag and goitre (either diffuse, e.g. Graves' disease, or nodular; note that goitre may be associated with hyper-, hypo- and euthyroid states). Graves' disease is associated with additional signs:

1. **Exophthalmos, i.e. protruding eyes; proptosis refers to eyes protruding beyond the orbit.**

2. **Ophthalmoplegia, i.e. paralysis of extraocular muscles causing strabismus (squint), as a result of muscle swelling and fibrosis. The patient will complain of diplopia (double vision).**

3. **Conjunctival oedema.**

4. **Periorbital oedema.**

5. **Pretibial myxoedema, i.e. painless thickening of skin in nodules or plaques over the shins.**

6. **Thyroid acropathy, i.e. clubbing.**

ⓘ Graves' disease is the most common cause of thyrotoxicosis, causing relapsing and remitting hyperthyroidism that often eventually progresses to hypothyroidism. It is associated with other autoimmune conditions such as pernicious anaemia, vitiligo, type 1 diabetes, coeliac disease and myasthenia gravis.

ⓘ Other causes of thyrotoxicosis include toxic adenoma (a single nodule that is 'hot' on scanning), toxic multinodular goitre (most common cause in elderly people), thyroiditis (transient hyperthyroidism resulting from acute inflammation of gland, e.g. post-viral (de Quervain's thyroiditis), metastatic thyroid cancer and drugs (e.g. excess T_4, amiodarone).

Q **What is the underlying cause of Graves' disease?** 2 marks

1. **TSH receptor IgG antibodies binding to the TSH receptor, which stimulate production of thyroid hormones.**

❶ These TSH receptor antibodies are not routinely measured, with the diagnosis of Graves' disease being made from the clinical features plus thyroid autoantibody measurement, i.e. autoantibodies against thyroglobulin and thyroid peroxidase. These autoantibodies may also occur in healthy individuals and those with Hashimoto's thyroiditis (see causes of *hypo*thyroidism).

Bloods are taken for TFTs as shown in the table.

Q **Indicate (↑, ↓ or ↔) where marked '?' for the expected changes** 3 marks

Hormone	Normal range	Hyperthyroidism	Hypothyroidism
TSH (mU/L)	0.5–5.7	↓	↑
Total T_4 (nmol/L)	70–140	↑	↓
Total T_3 (nmol/L)	1.2–3.0	↑	↓ ❶

❶ FT_4 and FT_3 are not routinely measured. However, several factors, including excess oestrogens, pregnancy, nephrotic syndrome and chronic liver disease, alter levels of TBG (and certain drugs also affect TBG binding), and as such total T_4 levels are inaccurate in these circumstances and so FT_4 should be measured to assess any thyrotoxicosis.

❶ Raised TSH with normal T_4 indicates subclinical hypothyroidism with treatment determined clinically. T_3 levels are often normal in hypothyroidism, reflecting upregulated peripheral conversion of T_4.

❶ Other investigations in hyperthyroidism may include erythrocyte sedimentation rate (ESR; increased in thyroiditis), thyroid ultrasonography to identify any solitary or multinodular goitre, and a radiolabelled iodine scan to assess thyroid uptake, i.e. 'hot' or 'cold' nodules. Thyroid malignancy usually presents as a 'cold' nodule (i.e. endocrinologically inactive) and is further investigated by fine-needle aspiration (FNA) or biopsy.

Endocrinology

163

Gloria's symptoms are treated with β blockers and her hyperthyroidism by 'block-and-replace' regimen with carbimazole and thyroxine.

Q Give one short-term and one long-term complication if her hyperthyroidism is untreated   **2 marks**

Short-term complication:

1. **Atrial fibrillation (AF): the risk of embolic stroke is high in AF associated with hyperthyroidism, and anticoagulation is mandatory.**

2. **Angina.**

3. **Thyrotoxic storm.**

Long-term complication:

1. **Osteoporosis.**

2. **Heart failure: causes thyrotoxic cardiomyopathy.**

❶ Treatment options for hyperthyroidism involve:

- Anti-thyroid drugs, e.g. carbimazole: can be either titrated up until adequate control or given in large doses to block the thyroid completely, with oral T_4 to keep the patient euthyroid. Propylthiouracil is an alternative. Measure TSH to monitor effectiveness of treatment.

- Radioactive iodine (iodine-131 or ^{131}I) therapy: single-dose treatment which is concentrated by the thyroid, causing cell death. The patient must stay away from pregnant women or young children for 17 days after the treatment. Patients usually end up hypothyroid, requiring lifelong thyroxine.

- Surgical resection (subtotal thyroidectomy) of the thyroid gland (see below).

❶ Thyroid crisis (thyrotoxic storm) is the result of a rapid deterioration of hyperthyroidism causing tachycardia, hyperthermia, confusion and coma. It may be triggered by myocardial infarction, trauma, infection, radioactive iodine or thyroid surgery (prevented by ensuring that the patient is euthyroid before surgery). Urgent treatment involves β blockers, potassium iodide, anti-thyroid drugs and corticosteroids.

❶ The eye problems of Graves' disease are typically independent of the thyroid status and are therefore not prevented by treating the hyperthyroidism (in fact, radioactive iodine therapy can transiently worsen the eye disease). Treatment may involve taping eyelids closed at night, lubricating eyedrops, lateral tarsorraphy (to protect the cornea), high-dose corticosteroids, orbital radiotherapy and occasionally surgical decompression of the orbit.

Q **Give four indications for thyroidectomy in Gloria**　　　　2 marks

1. **Patient choice, e.g. for cosmetic reasons.**

2. **Pressure symptoms from a large goitre, e.g. dyspnoea, dysphagia.**

3. **Intolerable drug side effects, e.g. carbimazole may cause agranulocytosis (propylthiouracil may also cause marrow suppression).**

4. **Poor compliance with drug therapy.**

5. **Relapse of hyperthyroidism after withdrawal of medication (patients are usually treated for 12–18 months).**

❶ In nodular goitre a further indication for surgery is the risk of thyroid cancer in these patients.

Q **Give four complications of surgery**　　　　2 marks

1. **Early postoperative bleeding causing dyspnoea as a result of haematoma pressure effects.**

2. **Hypothyroidism.**

3. **Recurrent hyperthyroidism.**

4. **Hypoparathyroidism causing hypocalcaemia (as a result of damage to adjacent parathyroid glands).**

5. **Hoarseness caused by recurrent laryngeal nerve damage.**

On cessation of the 'block-and-replace' regimen Gloria remains hyperthyroid. She is subsequently treated with radioactive iodine, which initially renders her euthyroid, although eventually it leaves her hypothyroid.

Q List four other causes of hypothyroidism 4 marks

1. Autoimmune hypothyroidism, e.g. Hashimoto's thyroiditis (causes a goitre; may be hypo-, hyper- or euthyroid), atrophic hypothyroidism (basically Hashimoto's thyroiditis without the goitre). Anti-thyroglobulin and anti-thyroid peroxidase antibodies may be present as well as anti-TSH receptor antibodies (although inhibitory as opposed to stimulatory).

2. Iodine deficiency: main cause of goitre and hypothyroidism worldwide.

3. Thyroidectomy or radioactive iodine treatment.

4. Drugs, e.g. anti-thyroid drugs, amiodarone.

5. Congenital (cretinism): screened for by the Guthrie heel-prick test at postnatal day 7 (detects increased TSH in heel-prick sample). The Guthrie test also detects phenylketonuria.

❶ Patients with symptomatic hypothyroidism require T_4; the aim of therapy is to return T_4 and TSH levels to normal (avoiding suppression of TSH). A dose of 100–150 µg/day is effective in most patients, although in patients with ischaemic heart disease they need to start at 25 µg/day and slowly titrate up to euthyroid levels.

❶ Amiodarone is an iodine-containing anti-arrhythmic that can cause either hyper- or hypothyroidism. In all patients it reduces the peripheral conversion of T_4 to T_3 so that T_4 levels may be raised without symptoms of hyperthyroidism (T_3 levels are low–normal). It can cause thyrotoxicosis by either destructive thyroiditis or iodine-induced excessive thyroid hormone synthesis (or conversely it may cause hypothyroidism).

Total **20 marks**

ENDOCRINOLOGY CASE 2

Jenny, a 21-year-old woman with type 1 diabetes, is seen by her GP after a 2-day history of nausea and vomiting; now she is complaining of abdominal pain. Urine dipstick showed glycosuria and ketonuria, and she is admitted to the medical assessment unit. On examination her GCS is 15/15, HR 120/min, abdomen tender throughout, and she is hyperventilating and appears to be dehydrated.

Q How is DKA diagnosed biochemically? 3 marks

1. **Hyperglycaemia: blood glucose typically > 20 mmol/L.**

2. **Ketonuria.**

3. **Acidosis: blood pH < 7.35.**

❶ DKA is caused by hyperglycaemia secondary to insulin deficiency, which causes osmotic diuresis resulting in dehydration; deficiency of intracellular glucose switches energy production to lipolysis, which forms ketone bodies (detected as ketonuria) and causes metabolic acidosis (associated with abdominal pain, which may be misdiagnosed as an acute abdomen, and vomiting, further exacerbating fluid and electrolyte balance). A diagnosis of DKA requires all three biochemical changes to be present.

Q List three causes of DKA 3 marks

1. **Presentation of type 1 diabetes**

2. **Interruption of insulin therapy, e.g. non-compliance.**

3. **Infection.**

4. **Surgery/trauma.**

5. **Myocardial infarction.**

QUESTIONS PAGES 24–26

❶ Although type 1 diabetes typically presents with the classic symptoms of polyuria, polydipsia, weight loss and lethargy, type 1 diabetes may also present with DKA.

❶ Examples 3–5 can cause DKA as a result of stress increasing insulin demand. The most common cause is for patients to reduce or omit insulin because they are unable to eat as a result of nausea and vomiting; all patients receive illness rules to minimise the risk of DKA (see below). Relevant investigations to identify the underlying cause include septic screen (chest radiograph, urine/blood cultures) and ECG.

❶ DKA is not associated with type 2 diabetes which may, however, cause hyperosmolar non-ketotic (HONK) coma: severe hyperglycaemia (> 35 mmol/L) but no acidosis/ketones. Treatment is essentially the same as DKA, i.e. less aggressive intravenous fluids and insulin.

Jenny is diagnosed with DKA. Her ABGs are shown below.

Q **Indicate (↑, ↓ or ↔) where marked '?' for the expected changes**   **4 marks**

	Normal range	Jenny's ABGs	Explanation
pH	7.35–7.45	↓	Acidosis caused by ketonaemia
Po_2 (kPa)	10–12	11	Depending on whether patient is shocked, hypoxia may or may not be present
Pco_2 (kPa)	4.7–6	↓	Hypocapnia as a result of respiratory compensation causing hyperventilation (Kussmaul's respiration or air hunger)
HCO_3^- (mmol/L)	22–28	↓	Bicarbonate depleted, attempting to buffer metabolic acidosis
BE (mmol/L)	±2	−9	Base deficit caused by HCO_3^- depletion
Anion gap	10–18	↑	Increased as a result of addition of 'unmeasured' ketones

Q **How do you calculate the anion gap?**   **1 mark**

1. **$(Na^+ + K^+) - (HCO_3^- + Cl^-)$.**

❶ The anion gap (AG) is calculated from the difference between plasma cations ($Na^+ + K^+$) and plasma anions ($HCO_3^- + Cl^-$); normal range is 10–18 mmol/L. ABG machines will calculate the AG for you.

168

❶ This is just an approximation because there are additional 'unmeasured' cations (e.g. calcium, magnesium) and anions (e.g. albumin, lactate); the total (Σ) unmeasured anions > Σ unmeasured cations, so there appears to be a positive anion gap (i.e. Σ cations > Σ anions), whereas in fact there is a state of electroneutrality (i.e. Σ cations = Σ anions).

Q **List three causes of metabolic acidosis with an *increased* anion gap** 3 marks

1. **Lactic acid, e.g. shock, sepsis.**

2 **Renal failure: as a result of accumulation of sulphate, urate, phosphate.**

3. **Ketones, e.g. DKA, alcohol, starvation.**

4. **Drugs, e.g. aspirin, metformin, methanol.**

❶ The AG is used to help identify the underlying cause of the metabolic acidosis. In metabolic acidosis with an increased AG there must be more 'unmeasured' anions, i.e. anions associated with acids.

❶ If the AG is normal metabolic acidosis is the result of either H^+ retention (e.g. type 1 renal tubular acidosis) or HCO_3^- loss (e.g. type 2 renal tubular acidosis, diarrhoea). In these conditions plasma bicarbonate is reduced and replaced by chloride to maintain electroneutrality.

❶ Bicarbonate is not routinely used in the treatment of DKA (it worsens intracellular acidosis), but is reserved for severe metabolic acidosis (pH < 7) not responding to treatment.

Jenny is successfully treated with intravenous fluids and intravenous insulin.

Q **List three complications of this treatment**   3 marks

1. **Fluid overload: this may cause pulmonary (and rarely cerebral) oedema.**

2. **Hypoglycaemia.**

3. **Hypokalaemia.**

❶ DKA typically presents with a fluid deficit of 5–12 L (less in those with an omitted insulin dose). Dehydration is more life threatening than hyperglycaemia and takes precedence. A typical regimen involves: 1.5 L in first hour, 1 L in next hour, 1 L in next 2 h, 2 L in next 8 h and then 0.5 L every 4 h, although reduced doses may be required in elderly/heart failure patients to avoid fluid overload.

❶ Initially, rehydration is with physiological (normal) saline (0.9 per cent) but, once blood glucose < 15 mmol/L, switch to 0.45 per cent saline + 5 per cent dextrose to prevent hypoglycaemia. The aim of intravenous insulin therapy is to reduce blood glucose by 3–4 mmol/h; initially give 4–6 units/h and then reduce to 3 units/h once glucose < 15 mmol/L (subsequently adjust insulin to maintain glucose between 5 and 10 mmol/ L). If higher rates of insulin infusion are required, it suggests an underlying cause such as sepsis or myocardial infarction.

❶ DKA patients are potassium deplete although initial plasma levels may be high/normal in response to the acidosis (as a result of cellular exchange of K^+ for H^+). Potassium levels decrease with rehydration (dilutional) and insulin (which drives potassium into the cells) and require replacement (usually with the second or third litres of fluid) and careful monitoring (as may cause arrhythmias).

❶ Once the patient is eating and drinking normally and there is no ketonuria, re-start the normal insulin regimen and take down the insulin infusion after the same meal. It is important to ensure that there is an overlap between re-starting subcutaneous insulin and stopping intravenous insulin to prevent rebound hyperglycaemia. In patients on once daily, long-acting insulin to cover basal insulin requirements (e.g. glargine) plus short-acting insulin with meals (e.g. NovoMix), a longer-acting insulin will be required (e.g. Actrapid) until the long-acting insulin is given (usually at night).

Once stabilised Jenny is referred to the diabetic nurse specialist for advice on the management of her diabetes.

Endocrinology

Q **List four 'illness rules' that you would give Jenny**   **2 marks**

1. **Obtain early treatment for infections.**

2. **Always take your insulin therapy.**

3. **Self-monitor more often during illnesses and adjust therapy accordingly (or seek advice if hyperglycaemic).**

4. **If unable to eat (e.g. anorexia, nauseous) take sweet fluids in place of meals.**

5. **Take plenty of sugar free fluids frequently to prevent dehydration.**

❶ Infections, caused by the increased stress on the body, increase insulin demand and may lead to a loss of glycaemic control, potentially causing DKA. This may be exacerbated by the common misconception that, if the patient is not eating properly, there is no need to take insulin.

Q **List four warning signs of hypoglycaemia**   **2 marks**

1. **Autonomic: sweating, palpitations, shaking, hunger.**

2. **Neurological: confusion, drowsiness, incoordination, odd behaviour, slurred speech.**

❶ The brain depends on a constant supply of glucose to maintain function; concentrations < 3.5 mmol/L impair neurological function. This activates the sympathetic nervous system, which opposes the actions of insulin and warns the patient. Risk is increased by missed meals and unusual exertion. All patients with type 1 diabetes should carry rapidly absorbed carbohydrate and a warning card.

Q **What two coexisting conditions should you screen for in Jenny?**   **2 marks**

1. **Hyper- and hypothyroidism: excluded by TFTs.**

2. **Coeliac disease: excluded by anti-gliadin antibody screen.**

❶ Type 1 diabetes, an autoimmune disease, is associated with thyroid and coeliac disease, the presence of which complicates good glycaemic control. These should be screened for at diagnosis and regular intervals throughout life.

171

Q List two challenges facing Jenny   **2 marks**

❶ There are no 'correct' answers to this question. However, it has been included to highlight the fact that diabetes is a self-managed disease and, if the patient is unwilling or unable to self-manage his or her own diabetes, the outcome is poor. The greatest barrier to good self-management is the challenges posed by diabetes, which may be specific to diabetes or to chronic diseases in general. A few examples are shown:

- **Managing medical treatment: regular blood tests and self-injecting, for example, may stigmatise the patient.**

- **Fear about the future: both short term, e.g. regular blood tests, and long term, e.g. blindness and complications of diabetes.**

- **The need for regular meals takes away spontaneity.**

Total   **25 marks**

GASTROINTESTINAL
CASES: ANSWERS

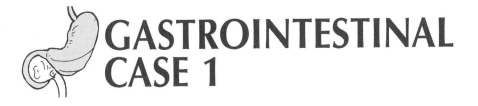

GASTROINTESTINAL CASE 1

Henry, a 58-year-old man, presents to A&E with a 1-hour history of haematemesis, including a severe episode in the ambulance. On examination his BP is 86/44 mmHg, he is cold peripherally and his pulse is 110 beats/min.

Q List six causes of haematemesis   **3 marks**

1. **Peptic ulcer disease (PUD).**

2. **Oesophageal varices.**

3. **Oesophagitis.**

4. **Gastritis.**

5. **Mallery–Weiss (oesophageal) tear: caused by excessive vomiting, e.g. as a result of alcohol, chemotherapy.**

6. **Upper GI malignancy, e.g. gastric cancer.**

7. **Arteriovenous malformations (AVMs).**

❶ The two main causes of PUD, which encompasses duodenal and gastric ulcers, are NSAIDs and *Helicobacter pylori* infection (see below).

❶ Portal hypertension, e.g. as a result of liver cirrhosis, causes dilated collateral veins (varices) at sites of portosystemic anastomosis, e.g. oesophagus, umbilicus (caput medusae), rectum and stomach. Those at the oesophagus may rupture, causing variceal bleeding; this is prevented by prophylactic β blockers, which lower portal hypertension.

Q What is your immediate management?   **3 marks**

QUESTIONS PAGES 29–31

ⓘ ABC as the patient is shocked, i.e. heart rate > systolic BP is a good working definition:

1. **Airways: protect airways by managing in recovery position.**

2. **Breathing: give high-flow O$_2$.**

3. **Circulation: obtain intravenous access with two large-bore cannulae and resuscitate with intravenous colloid/crystalloid while waiting for blood to be cross-matched (in emergencies can give O rhesus-negative blood).**

ⓘ Patients who are shocked and actively bleeding will require transfusion. Blood is also transfused if the Hb < 10 g/dL, to avoid adverse cardiovascular effects. However, massive transfusions can also cause coagulopathy requiring additional platelet and fresh frozen plasma (FFP) transfusions.

Q What three brief questions would you ask?   3 marks

1. **Any previous episodes of haematemesis and/or melaena (both indicate upper GI bleeds). including their cause, severity and treatment.**

2. **Any known causes of upper GI bleeds, e.g. PUD, chronic liver disease.**

3. **Any dyspeptic symptoms, e.g. epigastric pain, gastro-oesophageal reflux disease (GORD).**

4. **Alcohol consumption, intravenous drug use (IVDU): alcohol, and hepatitis B and C virus (from IVDU) are the main causes of liver cirrhosis.**

5. **Medication history, e.g. NSAIDs, aspirin, warfarin.**

ⓘ Examination should include rectal examination (for melaena) and search for signs (stigmata) of chronic liver disease.

Q What four blood tests would you request?   2 marks

1. **Full blood count (FBC): anaemia (Hb may not fall until circulating volume is restored), thrombocytopenia (increased risk of bleeding).**

2. **U&Es (urea and electrolytes): any electrolyte abnormalities.**

3. **Clotting screen: any bleeding disorder, e.g. ↑ INR (international normalised ratio).**

4. **Liver function tests (LFTs): suspect varices if chronic liver disease; liver disease causes increased INR as a result of reduced clotting factor synthesis and reduced vitamin K absorption (fat-soluble vitamin requiring bile for absorption).**

5. **Group and save (G&S)/cross-match: if active bleeding cross-match 4–6 units.**

❶ In the presence of a bleeding disorder, consult a haematologist for advice on vitamin K injection, FFP and platelet transfusion.

❶ Endoscopy (OGD) should be performed within 24 hours or within 4 hours in the presence of active bleeding or if a variceal haemorrhage is suspected. Endoscopy has three purposes: (1) diagnosis, (2) prognosis (see below) and (3) treatment, e.g. banding of varices or epinephrine injection into bleeding ulcers.

❶ If a variceal haemorrhage is confirmed on endoscopy (or suspected in bleeding associated with stigmata of liver disease) give intravenous terlipressin (antidiuretic hormone [ADH] derivative), which constricts the splanchnic artery and restricts portal inflow. If there is severe or continuous variceal bleeding, pass a Sengstaken–Blakemore tube to compress oesophageal varices (this should be attempted by your senior).

Henry undergoes emergency endoscopy, which diagnoses an actively bleeding gastric ulcer; this is successfully treated by an injection of epinephrine.

Q What factors are used to assess Henry's risk of re-bleeding   **4 marks**

1. **Age.**

2. **Shock.**

3. **Co-morbidity: death after an upper GI bleed is usually a result of decompensated co-morbidity rather than exsanguination.**

4. **Endoscopic findings: presence of blood in the upper GI tract, active spurting haemorrhage and non-bleeding visible vessels are all poor prognostic signs.**

● It is important to identify those patients at risk of continuing bleeding or re-bleeding because they will require more intensive monitoring (see below). The Rockhall score is used to predict those at risk of re-bleeding and death; a score > 6 is high risk.

Rockhall risk scoring system

Score	0	1	2	3
Age (years)	< 60	60–79	80	–
Shock Systolic BP (mmHg) Pulse (/min)	None	 > 100 > 100	 < 100 	–
Co-morbidity	None	–	Cardiac or other major disease	Renal or liver failure; malignancy
Diagnosis on OGD	None Mallory–Weiss tear No sign of recent bleeding	All other diagnoses	Upper GI malignancy	–
Signs of recent haemorrhage	None Black spots	–	Blood in upper GI tract Clot Spurting haemorrhage Non-bleeding visible vessel	–

Q **List four signs of a re-bleed while on the ward**   2 marks

1. **Increasing heart rate.**

2. **Decreasing blood pressure.**

3. **Decreasing central venous pressure (although not all patients will have a central line).**

Gastrointestinal

4. **Decreasing hourly urine output: patients should be catheterised so urinary output can be monitored.**

5. **Haematemesis.**

6. **Melaena.**

❶ Management after re-bleeding usually involves repeat endoscopy. Surgery, e.g. ulcer excision, is indicated when active bleeding cannot be controlled by endoscopy therapy (either at presentation or after re-bleeding) or exsanguinating haemorrhage (i.e. too fast to replace or requiring > 6 units blood to restore blood pressure); as such warn surgeon on call of all serious non-variceal bleeds.

❶ To prevent re-bleeding in high-risk cases start intravenous omeprazole infusion, i.e. 80 mg bolus followed by 8 mg/h for 72 h (clot formation is impaired in an acid environment).

Henry's rapid urease test on endoscopy confirms H. pylori *infection and the endoscopist recommends triple therapy for eradication and avoidance of NSAIDs.*

Q What does this regimen involve? 1 mark

1. **This involves 1 week's treatment with:**

- **A proton pump inhibitor (PPI), e.g. omeprazole 20 mg twice daily.**

- **Amoxicillin: 1 g twice daily.**

- **Clarithromycin (500 mg twice daily) or metronidazole (400 mg three times daily).**

❶ This achieves eradication in over 90 per cent of cases. If the patient does not have an ulcer, no continuing treatment is required; if the patient does have an ulcer he or she should continue the PPI (once daily) for 6 weeks.

❶ H. pylori infection can be detected on endoscopy (e.g. rapid urease test, histology, culture) and non-invasive tests (e.g. carbon-13 [^{13}C] urea breath test, serology). Serology for H. pylori antibodies cannot be used after treatment.

179

Q Name two drugs used to reduce GI side effects of NSAIDs   **2 marks**

❶ NSAIDs inhibit cyclo-oxygenase (COX), which exists in two isoforms: (1) COX-1 is constitutively expressed in many tissues and inhibition causes loss of gastric mucosal protection, and (2) COX-2 is induced in response to inflammation. Ideally NSAIDs should be stopped after an upper GI haemorrhage, although in patients who require continuing NSAID therapy the GI side effects can be reduced by:

1. **Selective COX-2 inhibitor.**

2. **Non-selective NSAID + PPI.**

3. **Non-selective NSAID + misoprostol (prostaglandin analogue).**

❶ There is no evidence that COX-2 inhibitors plus a gastroprotective drug further reduce the GI side effects.

Total   **20 marks**

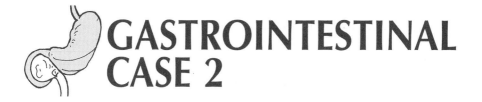

GASTROINTESTINAL CASE 2

Rod, a 48-year-old man, is admitted to the medical assessment unit complaining of malaise and anorexia. On examination he is jaundiced with signs of chronic liver disease.

Q List four risk factors for jaundice that you would enquire about in the *social* history   **2 marks**

1. **IVDU: increased risk of hepatitis B and C viruses (HBV, HCV).**

2. **Tattoos: increased risk of HBV and HCV.**

3. **Excessive alcohol consumption: alcoholic liver disease.**

4. **Homosexuality: increased risk of HBV.**

5. **Health-care worker: increased risk of HBV and HCV.**

6. **Farm or sewage worker: increased risk of leptospira infection.**

7. **Water sports: increased risk of leptospira infection.**

8. **Recent travel abroad: to areas endemic for hepatitis A virus (HAV). (However hepatitis A does not usually cause chronic liver disease)**

❶ It is also important in the history to enquire about medications (e.g. statins, anti-tuberculosis [anti-TB]) and obstructive symptoms, i.e. pale stools and dark urine.

❶ Jaundice can be classified as:

- Prehepatic (unconjugated hyperbilirubinaemia): as a result of haemolysis, impaired hepatic uptake and reduced conjugation (caused by impaired glucuronyl transferase activity).

- Hepatocellular: hepatocyte damage ± intrahepatic cholestasis.

- Cholestatic (obstructive): intra- and extrahepatic cholestasis.

**QUESTIONS
PAGES
32–34**

❶ Extrahepatic causes of obstructive jaundice include gallstones, pancreatic cancer, benign stricture of the common bile duct (e.g. complication of endoscopic retrograde cholangiopancreatography [ERCP]), sclerosing cholangitis (e.g. associated with IBD) and cholangiocarcinoma.

Q List three *abdominal* signs of chronic liver disease   3 marks

1. **Hepatomegaly (or small liver in late disease).**

2. **Ascites (see below).**

3. **Splenomegaly: caused by portal hypertension.**

4. **Caput medusa (dilated collateral veins around the umbilicus): resulting from portal hypertension.**

❶ Other signs of chronic liver disease include: hands (clubbing, palmar erythema, leukonychia, Dupuytren's contracture), endocrine disturbances (loss of body hair, testicular atrophy, gynaecomastia), peripheral oedema (caused by hypoalbuminaemia) and spider naevi (occur on upper body in the drainage of the superior vena cava [SVC]; five or more suggest liver disease).

❶ Liver failure may occur in a previously healthy liver (i.e. acute liver failure) or after decompensation of chronic liver disease (acute-on-chronic liver failure). Fulminant hepatic failure refers to hepatic encephalopathy (see below) in the context of acute liver failure.

Several blood tests are requested to assess the severity of Rod's liver failure.

Q Name two blood tests used to assess liver synthetic function   2 marks

❶ There are only two tests of liver synthetic function:

1. **Albumin (normal range 35–50 g/L): hypoalbuminaemia typically reflects chronic liver disease. The resulting reduction in plasma oncotic pressure promotes peripheral oedema and ascites.**

2. **INR (normal range 0.9–1.2)/prothrombin time (PT – normal range 10–14 s): increased as a result of impaired synthesis of clotting factors and vitamin K malabsorption (fat-soluble vitamin requiring bile).**

❶ Other blood tests used to assess liver disease are:

1. FBC: reduced white cell count (WCC) and reduced platelets indicate hypersplenism.

2. U&Es, e.g. hyponatraemia caused by secondary hyperaldosteronism (aldosterone is normally metabolised by the liver).

3. LFTs: may get raised AST (aspartate transaminase), ALT (alanine transaminase), ALP (alkaline phosphatase), GGT (γ-glutamyl transferase) and bilirubin.

4. Glucose: hypoglycaemia.

❶ LFTs do not actually assess liver function; they are non-specific indicators of liver or biliary disease. For example, raised AST and ALT reflect hepatocellular damage whereas raised ALP and GGT reflect cholestasis (either intra- or extrahepatic).

Abdominal ultrasonography reports cirrhotic changes in the liver (later confirmed on liver biopsy) with gross ascites.

Q **In the absence of obvious risk factors list six blood tests that you would request to identify the cause of Rod's liver cirrhosis** 3 marks

1. **FBC: raised mean corpuscular volume (MCV), i.e. macrocytosis, is an indicator of alcohol misuse.**

2. **Hepatitis B and C virus serology.**

3. **α_1-Antitrypsin level: to exclude α_1-antitrypsin deficiency.**

4. **Copper studies (reduced serum copper and ceruloplasmin, a copper-containing protein synthesised by the liver): to exclude Wilson's disease which results in copper deposition in the liver.**

5. **Iron studies (increased iron and ferritin, and reduced total iron-binding capacity [TIBC]: to exclude haemochromatosis resulting in iron deposition in the liver.**

6. **Autoantibodies: used to identify autoimmune causes of cirrhosis: anti-mitochondrial antibody (AMA; primary biliary cirrhosis [PBC]), anti-nuclear antibody (ANA) and smooth muscle antibody (SMA; autoimmune hepatitis).**

❶ Chronic liver disease may progress to cirrhosis as a result of irreversible liver damage. This is confirmed on liver biopsy; histologically, there is fibrotic and nodular regeneration with loss of normal hepatic architecture.

❶ The severity of liver cirrhosis is based on the Child–Pugh grading:

Score	1 point	2 points	3 points
Bilirubin (μmol/L)	< 34	34–51	> 51
Albumin (g/L)	> 35	28-35	< 28
PT (s) (> normal)	1–4	4–6	> 6
Ascites	None	Slight	Moderate
Encephalopathy[a]	None	Grade 1–2	Grade 3–4

[a]For grading of encephalopathy: see below
Grading of cirrhosis: grade A < 7, grade B7–9 and grade C > 9.

It is apparent from Rod's social history that the cause of his liver failure is alcoholic liver disease and he is given intravenous thiamine and started on chlordiazepoxide-reducing regimen.

Q Why do we give thiamine to people with alcohol problems?　　1 mark

1. To prevent Wernicke–Korsakoff syndrome.

❶ Thiamine (vitamin B_1) deficiency in people with alcohol problems may cause Wernicke's encephalopathy, characterised by ophthalmoplegia, ataxia and confusion, which if not treated may progress to irreversible Korsakoff's syndrome. This causes anterograde amnesia, resulting in confabulation, i.e. making up stories to fill in the gaps in memory.

❶ All patients with alcohol problems should be given an intravenous thiamine (Pabrinex) and chlordiazepoxide (Librium) reducing regimen (to relieve the symptoms of withdrawal). Thiamine must be given before any intravenous glucose infusion because this may precipitate Wernicke's encephalopathy.

❶ Thiamine deficiency (e.g. those with alcohol problems, malnutrition, persistent vomiting) may also cause *dry beri-beri* (peripheral neuropathy) and *wet beri-beri* (peripheral oedema).

Gastrointestinal

Q How would you treat Rod's ascites? 3 marks

1. **Fluid restriction: < 1.5 L/day.**

2. **Low salt diet: < 0.5 g/day.**

3. **Spironolactone (aldosterone antagonist): start with 50 mg twice daily and titrate up to 200–400 mg/day (± furosemide if no response). Diuretics should be temporarily discontinued if creatinine starts rising, representing over-diuresis and hypovolaemia.**

❶ Ascites, i.e. accumulation of fluid in the peritoneal cavity, indicates a poor prognosis in chronic liver disease and may be demonstrated by shifting dullness or a fluid thrill. It is caused by a combination of splanchnic vasodilatation, resulting in sodium and water retention (exacerbated by secondary hyperaldosteronism), and portal hypertension forcing transudation of fluid into the peritoneal cavity (exacerbated by hypoalbuminaemia).

❶ Refractory or symptomatic tense ascites can be drained (therapeutic paracentesis) with concomitant albumin infusion (8 g/L fluid removed – use human albumin 20 per cent not the standard 4.5 per cent bottles) to help prevent hypovolaemia because ascites reaccumulates at the expense of circulating volume.

❶ Avoid saline infusions in patients with ascites; use 5 per cent dextrose for fluid maintenance.

Several days later Rod starts to deteriorate, complaining of severe abdominal pain. On examination his abdomen is very tender with guarding and he is pyrexial.

Q What is the likely complication? 2 marks

1. **Spontaneous bacterial peritonitis (SBP).**

❶ Spontaneous bacterial peritonitis is a serious complication (25 per cent mortality rate), affecting approximately 10 per cent of cirrhotic ascites. It should be suspected in any patient with clinical deterioration even in the absence of abdominal pain and pyrexia.

Gastrointestinal

Q How would you confirm your diagnosis?   1 mark

1. Aspirate ascitic fluid for urgent MC&S.

❶ A WCC > 250/mm³ in aspirated ascitic fluid is considered diagnostic of bacterial peritonitis. It is treated with antibiotics, e.g. ciprofloxacin 500 mg twice daily.

Q List three additional complications of liver cirrhosis   3 marks

1. Renal failure (hepatorenal syndrome): caused by compensatory renal vasoconstriction in response to peripheral vasodilatation (due to nitric oxide), resulting in a reduced glomerular filtration rate that causes pre-renal failure or acute tubular necrosis.

2. Hepatic encephalopathy: caused by 'toxic metabolites' (e.g. ammonia) in the blood bypassing the liver by portosystemic collaterals, resulting in neurotoxicity.

3. Portal hypertension: causes variceal haemorrhage (see Gastrointestinal case 1), hypersplenism.

4. Coagulopathy (see above): treatment involves vitamin K 10 mg i.v. (± FFP if bleeding).

5. Hepatocellular carcinoma: screen by regular ultrasonography and α-fetoprotein (AFP).

❶ Hepatic encephalopathy can occur acutely or chronically. It is graded as follows:

Grade	Symptoms and signs
1	Altered mood or behaviour
2	Confusion, drowsy
3	Stupor, incoherence, agitation
4	Coma

ⓘ Other features include fetor hepaticus (pear drop breath), constructional apraxia (e.g. unable to draw five-point star) and coarse flapping tremor (when arms outstretched and wrists hyperextended). Acute encephalopathy often has a precipitating factor, e.g. constipation, infection, drugs (e.g. central nervous system [CNS] depressants), electrolyte disturbance (e.g. secondary to diuretics or GI bleed). Management involves correction of the underlying cause, e.g. lactulose, antibiotics, stopping diuretic therapy.

Total   **20 marks**

Gastrointestinal

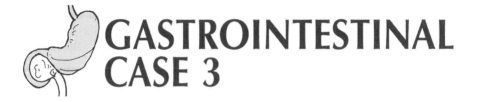

GASTROINTESTINAL CASE 3

Dennis, a 64-year-old man, is admitted to the surgical assessment unit with a history of severe epigastric pain, radiating to his back, of several hours associated with nausea and vomiting. His serum amylase is reported as 670 U/mL (normal range 0–180 U/mL), confirming a diagnosis of acute pancreatitis.

Q List eight criteria used to assess the severity of pancreatitis　　　**4 marks**

	Criteria	Positive value	Normal range
P	**Po₂** (kPa)	< 8	> 10.6
A	**Age** (years)	> 55	
N	**Neutrophils** (× 10⁹/L)	WCC > 15	4–11
C	**Calcium (adjusted)** (mmol/L)	< 2	2.12–2.65
R	**Renal function** (mmol/L)	Urea > 16	2.5–6.7
E	**Enzymes**		70–250
	LDH (IU/L)	> 600	3–35
	AST (IU/L)	> 200	
A	**Albumin** (g/L)	< 32	35–50
S	**Sugar (blood glucose)** (mmol/L)	> 10	4–6

❶ Acute pancreatitis is diagnosed on the basis of clinical features and confirmed by serum amylase levels more than three times the upper limit of normal. However, amylase levels decline over 2–3 days so a normal amylase does not exclude pancreatitis in patients with symptoms for more than 3 days (amylase is also elevated in non-pancreatic conditions, e.g. visceral perforation, small bowel obstruction or ischaemia, leaking aortic aneurysm, ectopic pregnancy).

QUESTIONS
PAGES
35–37

❶ The Glasgow scoring system is used to predict the severity of acute pancreatitis from both gallstones and alcohol (Ranson's criteria are valid for alcohol-induced pancreatitis only). Three or more positive criteria indicate severe pancreatitis. Other predictors of a severe attack include obesity (body mass index > 30), pleural effusion on chest radiograph and raised C-reactive protein (CRP > 150 mg/L).

❶ The purpose of predicting severity is to identify those patients at high risk of complications and who should be managed on intensive care. Early complications include shock (see below), acute renal failure, acute respiratory distress syndrome (ARDS), disseminated intravascular coagulation (DIC) and metabolic complications (e.g. hyperglycaemia, hypocalcaemia); late complications include pancreatic necrosis and pseudocyst (fluid in lesser sac).

Q **List three causes of acute pancreatitis** 3 marks

1. **Gallstones (50 per cent).**

2. **Alcohol (20 per cent): may represent an exacerbation of chronic pancreatitis as opposed to true acute pancreatitis.**

3. **Idiopathic (20 per cent).**

4. **Drugs (5 per cent), e.g. steroids, furosemide, azathioprine.**

5. **Viral infection, e.g. HIV, mumps.**

6. **Hypertriglyceridaemia.**

7. **ERCP.**

❶ Gallstones can cause acute pancreatitis by blocking the hepatopancreatic ampulla, resulting in reflux back up the main pancreatic duct and leading to pancreatic autodigestion. Deranged LFTs on admission may indicate a biliary cause; all patients should have abdominal ultrasonography to look for gallstones and dilated bile ducts (early abdominal computed tomography is, however, unhelpful).

Dennis is kept NBM, given high-flow oxygen therapy and aggressive fluid replacement. A urinary catheter is inserted to monitor his urine output.

189

Q **In fluid replacement, what minimum hourly urinary output do you aim for?** 3 marks

1. Aim for urine flow > 30 mL/h (ideally should be 60 mL/h).

❶ Acute pancreatitis is (initially) managed conservatively with oxygen therapy and aggressive fluid resuscitation (colloid and crystalloid) to replace plasma volume deficit (as a result of third space fluid loss, i.e. extracellular fluid trapped in the gut, peritoneum and retroperitoneum) and maintain urine output (may also require central venous pressure monitoring).

❶ Patients are initially kept NBM with insertion of a nasogastric tube if there is protracted vomiting (resulting from small bowel ileus), although early enteral nutrition (e.g. via a nasogastric tube) is now recommended.

❶ Prophylactic antibiotics are indicated only in patients with pancreatic necrosis (see below). Pyrexia on presentation usually represents a non-infective systemic inflammatory response syndrome (SIRS) and does not warrant antibiotics (unless associated with cholangitis).

Dennis undergoes an abdominal ultrasound scan, which shows gallbladder stones with their acoustic shadows.

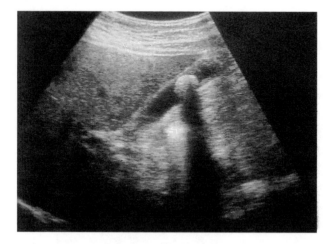

Q **Name six additional complications of gallstones** 3 marks

1. Biliary colic: caused by bile duct attempting to shift impacted gallstones.

2. **Cholecystitis (see below).**

3. **Empyema: obstructed gallbladder fills with pus.**

4. **Obstructive jaundice: resulting from gallstones obstructing the common bile duct (CBD).**

5. **Cholangitis: infection of the bile ducts causing right upper quadrant pain, jaundice and rigors (Charcot's triad).**

6. **Gallbladder perforation and generalised peritonitis.**

7. **Gallstone ileus: caused by gallstones obstructing the small bowel.**

❶ Acute cholecystitis is caused by gallstones obstructing the cystic duct, resulting in gallbladder distension (which may cause local peritonism) and (sterile) inflammation (raised WCC, fever). Presenting features include severe right upper quadrant (RUQ) pain with nausea, vomiting and sweating, and a positive Murphy sign. Murphy's sign is arrest of inspiration (caused by severe pain) on palpation just below the right subcostal margin, resulting from the inflamed gallbladder descending to touch your hand (only positive if same test on left-hand side is negative).

Q What is the recommended procedure within the first 72 hours? 2 marks

1. **ERCP ± sphincterotomy and removal of any stones.**

❶ All patients with severe pancreatitis associated with gallstones (with or without evidence of biliary obstruction) should have ERCP within 72 h. ERCP involves insertion of an endoscope into the second part of the duodenum, cannulating the ampula and injecting radio-opaque dye to visualise the biliary tree (an alternative imaging technique is magnetic resonance cholangiopancreatography). Any stone found on radiograph can be removed by sphincterotomy of the biliary sphincter and swept clear.

❶ Abdominal computed tomography (CT; contrast enhanced to detect necrosis) is usually performed in patients with severe pancreatitis (or with clinical deterioration) after 7–10 days for detection of pancreatic complications. FNA of pancreatic tissue may be indicated (e.g. necrosis associated with signs of sepsis) to diagnose infected necrosis, which is treated by radiological (drainage) or surgical (necrosectomy) intervention. Pseudocysts are drained only if symptomatic.

Gastrointestinal

Dennis undergoes a cholecystectomy before discharge.

Q **List two advantages each of laparoscopic and open cholecystectomy** 2 marks

1. **Laparoscopic: reduced wound pain, less scar formation, shorter in-patient stay/quicker recovery.**

2. **Open: lower risk of bile duct injury, lower risk of damage to adjacent structures, able simultaneously to remove any stones in the CBD, technically easier.**

❶ Patients with gallstone pancreatitis should have cholecystectomy, ideally during the same admission.

Q **Give three complications of cholecystectomy** 3 marks

1. **Death: < 1 per 1000.**

2. **Bile duct injury.**

3. **Bile leakage.**

4. **Jaundice resulting from retained ductal stones (can be removed by ERCP).**

5. **Wound infection.**

6. **General complications of any surgical procedure, e.g. pulmonary embolism, chest infection.**

Total 20 marks

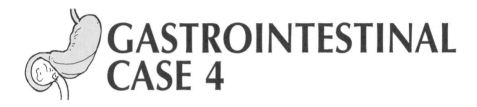

GASTROINTESTINAL CASE 4

Annie, a 25-year-old woman, presents with a 4-week history of diarrhoea with some mucus and blood mixed in her stool. She also complains of general abdominal discomfort, malaise and weight loss.

Q **List four causes of bloody diarrhoea**   **4 marks**

1. **Ulcerative colitis.**

2. **Crohn's disease: rectal bleeding is associated with colonic disease, although it is not as severe as UC.**

3. **Colorectal cancer.**

4. **Colonic polyps.**

5. **Ischaemic colitis: due to chronic ischaemia of the bowel.**

6. **Pseudomembranous colitis: caused by overgrowth of *Clostridium difficile* following antibiotic therapy.**

7. **Infective (dysentery): *Escherichia coli* O157, and *Shigella, Salmonella* and *Campylobacter* spp.**

❶ Although UC and Crohn's disease both cause diarrhoea and abdominal pain with systemic features such as malaise and weight loss, the hallmark of UC is bloody diarrhoea.

Q **Why would you do a plain abdominal radiograph in an acute attack of UC?**   **2 marks**

1. **To exclude toxic megacolon, i.e. colon diameter > 5.5 cm, which is associated with a high risk of perforation (see complications below)**

2. **To assess faecal distribution: the distal extent of constipation indicates how far UC extends proximally because affected bowel will be empty of stool (black with air).**

❶ Other investigations for UC include FBC (anaemia), vitamin B$_{12}$ (often low if terminal ileitis), U&Es (electrolyte imbalance as a result of diarrhoea), LFTs (may be deranged, albumin often low), ESR/CRP (severity of inflammation), stool and blood microscopy, culture and sensitivities (MC&S; to exclude infectious diarrhoea), and sigmoidoscopy. A barium enema or colonoscopy with biopsy to assess disease extent is contraindicated during an acute severe attack of UC as a result of the risk of perforation.

❶ In Crohn's disease the small bowel is imaged using barium follow-through (may show strictures, ulceration) and large bowel by barium enema (may show deep 'rose-thorn' ulceration and a cobblestone appearance as a result of widespread ulceration) ± colonoscopy.

Annie is given a phosphate enema and undergoes a sigmoidoscopy, which reveals a superficial continuous inflammation of the rectum. The mucosa looks reddened and inflamed, consistent with UC.

Q **List four pathological differences between UC and Crohn's disease**   **4 marks**

1. **UC involves only the bowel mucosa whereas Crohn's disease involves all layers of the bowel wall (transmural – this may lead to fistulas).**

2. **Crohn's disease causes skip lesions (normal areas of bowel in between).**

3. **Crohn's disease can affect any part of the GI tract (i.e. mouth to anus) but typically affects the terminal ileum and ascending colon.**

4. **UC can affect rectum alone (proctitis) but can also extend proximally to involve part or all of the colon (colitis); it rarely spreads proximally beyond the colon (termed 'backwash ileitis').**

❶ Surgery is curative of the intestinal features of UC and typically involves colectomy with an ileostomy or ileoanal pouch reconstruction. Indications for surgery include perforation, massive haemorrhage, toxic dilatation and failure to respond to medication. However, surgery is not curative in Crohn's disease because disease may recur anywhere in the GI tract, although most patients will require an operation, e.g. for fistulas, strictures.

Q List four extraintestinal manifestations of IBD
2 marks

Related to disease activity	Unrelated to disease activity
Mouth: aphthous ulcers	**Joints**: sacroiliitis, ankylosing spondylitis
Skin: pyoderma gangrenosum, erythema nodosum	**Liver**: primary sclerosing cholangitis, fatty liver, cirrhosis, cholangiocarcinoma, gallstones
Eyes: conjunctivitis, episcleritis, uveitis	Finger clubbing
Joints: acute arthritis	

❶ Extraintestinal manifestations occur in 10–20 per cent of patients, of which only some are related to disease activity. Colectomy does not cure ankylosing spondylitis or primary sclerosing cholangitis.

Q List six features used to assess the severity of UC
3 marks

Features	Mild	Moderate	Severe attack
Motions per day	< 4	4–6	> 6
Rectal bleeding	Little	Moderate	Large amounts
Temperature (°C)	Apyrexial	Intermediate	> 37.8
Pulse rate (beats/min)	< 70	70–90	> 90
Haemoglobin (g/dL)	> 11	10.5–11	< 10.5
ESR (mm/h)	Normal	Intermediate	> 30

❶ UC can be classified according to the above features as mild, moderate or severe, which is used to determine management. Mild and moderate attacks are treated with rectal (enemas or suppositories in patients with distal colitis or proctitis) and oral steroids. An alternative to oral steroids in mild UC is oral high-dose mesalazine (Pentasa).

❶ Severe attacks require admittance and treatment by intravenous fluids, potassium supplements (also consider total parenteral nutrition), intravenous and rectal steroids and, if necessary, blood transfusion. CRP > 45 mg/L and stool frequency of more than eight per day after 3 days of intravenous therapy is an indication for surgery. Do not give anti-diarrhoeal drugs because they increase the risk of perforation.

🛈 Severity in Crohn's disease is harder to assess than in UC. Treatment (in both acute attacks and long-term maintenance therapy) is similar to UC, although some attacks respond to elemental diets alone (which act to rest the bowel).

Annie is treated with oral and rectal steroids and responds well to treatment.

Q What class of drug is prescribed to maintain remission in UC?   **2 marks**

1. Aminosalicylates: the active ingredient is 5-aminosalicylic acid (5-ASA), e.g. mesalazine, olsalazine, sulfasalazine.

🛈 All patients with UC should be treated with aminosalicylates, which reduce the risk of relapse from 80 to 20 per cent within the first year; corticosteroids have no role in maintaining remission. Their mechanism of action is unclear; however, the preparations deliver 5-ASA to the site of action, usually the large bowel (via the actions of colonic bacteria) or distal ileum (pH-dependent release). A rare but serious side effect is blood dyscrasias (e.g. aplastic anaemia, neutropenia, thrombocytopenia, agranulocytosis).

🛈 5-ASA may also be given as a suppository (for proctitis) or enema (for distal colitis) during an acute attack.

🛈 Azathioprine is an immunosuppressant (inhibits DNA synthesis) that can be used as a steroid-sparing agent in those with severe steroid side effects or those with frequent relapses on withdrawal of steroids.

Q Give three complications of ulcerative colitis   **3 marks**

1. Perforation.

2. Bleeding: massive haemorrhage is rare.

3. Malnutrition.

4. **Toxic dilatation of the colon: this may occur during an acute severe attack of UC (and Crohn's disease). This should be expected in any patient developing abdominal distension and is diagnosed on abdominal radiograph by colon diameter > 5.5 cm. If not responding to high-dose steroids it may require emergency surgery because the risk of perforation is high.**

5. **Colon cancer: incidence of colon cancer is increased in UC (and less so in Crohn's disease). Risk is highest in those with extensive UC for > 10 years and such patients require monitoring with regular colonoscopy with multiple biopsies.**

❶ These complications also occur (more rarely) in Crohn's disease. More common complications in Crohn's disease include strictures (mainly affect small bowel), perianal disease (e.g. fissures, fistulas and abscesses) and fistulas, i.e. abnormal communication between bowel and bladder, vagina, and/or skin.

Total   **20 marks**

Gastrointestinal

NEUROLOGY CASES: ANSWERS

NEUROLOGY CASE 1

George, a 72-year-old man on treatment for hypertension, is admitted with a stroke. Examination reveals weakness, sensory loss and homonymous hemianopia on the affected side.

Q List two visual symptoms that George might be complaining of   **2 marks**

❶ Homonymous hemianopia causes loss of vision in the contralateral visual field with the result that patients complain of:

1. **Knocking into objects.**

2. **Seeing only half of objects, e.g. face, clock, plate of food.**

3. **Unable to read because sees only half the page.**

❶ Homonymous hemianopia is caused by lesions to the optic tract, optic radiation or visual cortex (macular vision may be spared), and may arise from occlusions to the middle cerebral artery (which supplies the optic radiation) or posterior cerebral artery (which supplies the occipital cortex).

Q Name two sensory modalities carried in the posterior column   **2 marks**

1. **Proprioception.**

2. **Vibration.**

3. **Discriminative touch.**

❶ Two major ascending pathways are involved in somatic sensory perception: (1) posterior column–medial lemniscal pathway and (2) spinothalamic pathway carrying pain, temperature and light touch.

? QUESTIONS
PAGES
43–45

❶ The corticospinal (or pyramidal) tracts project from the cerebral cortex, descend through the internal capsule, cross (decussate) in the medulla and descend in the lateral and anterior white columns of the spinal cord before synapsing with lower motor neurons in the anterior horn. After a stroke weak limbs are at first flaccid and areflexic, although eventually they become hypertonic (spastic) and hyperreflexive (upper motor neuron signs).

Q **Name four cardiac conditions that may cause an embolic stroke**   **4 marks**

❶ A stroke may be caused by haemorrhage (as a result of rupture of microaneurysms secondary to hypertension), local thrombus formation, atherothromboembolism (e.g. thrombus associated with atheroma in arterial supply to brain) or a heart embolus (the last three cause infarction by occluding the cerebral artery):

1. **Atrial fibrillation (AF).**

2. **Myocardial infarction causing a mural thrombus.**

3. **Infective endocarditis.**

4. **Aortic or mitral valve disease.**

5. **Patent foramen ovale (paradoxical embolus).**

6. **Cardiac tumours, e.g. left atrial myxoma.**

❶ When examining a stroke patient, it is necessary to identify (1) the neurological deficits by carrying out a full neurological examination, (2) factors that may cause complications, e.g. dysphagia, and (3) likely causes of the stroke, e.g. full cardiovascular system (CVS) examination to exclude AF, heart murmurs and carotid bruits.

Q **List six features associated with a lesion to the vertebrobasilar territory**   **3 marks**

❶ The neurological consequences of a stroke depend on the region of brain affected. Localisation requires knowledge of arterial blood supply to the brain (Figure 1) and location of different functions within the brain (Figure 2). A lesion to the vertebrobasilar territory, which supplies the brain stem and cerebellum, may cause:

Neurology

1. **Cranial nerve signs (resulting from brain-stem lesion), e.g. diplopia (cranial nerves [CNs] III, IV, VI), facial weakness (CN VII), facial numbness (CN V), vertigo (CN VIII), dysphagia (CNs IX and X) and dysarthria (CNs IX, X and XII).**

2. **Ataxia (resulting from lesion to cerebellum).**

3. **Weakness in both arms or legs (caused by lesion to corticospinal tracts).**

4. **Sensory loss in both arms or legs (caused by lesion to ascending sensory pathways).**

5. **Coma (resulting from lesion to reticular formation).**

6. **Locked-in syndrome, i.e. aware but unable to respond (caused by massive brain-stem lesion).**

❶ The lateral medullary syndrome (resulting from posteroinferior cerebellar artery lesion) causes vertigo, ataxia, and loss of pain and temperature on the ipsilateral face and contralateral limbs. There is no limb weakness because the corticospinal tracts are unaffected.

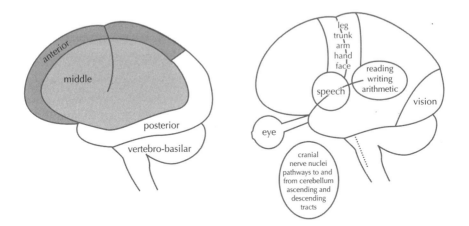

Figure 1 Arterial supply to the brain.   Figure 2 Functions of the brain.

George undergoes a number of investigations including CT of the brain.

203

George's brain CT scan is shown.

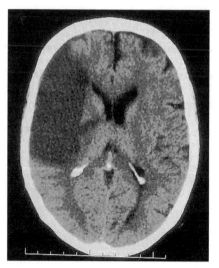

Q **Is George's stroke the result of an infarction or a haemorrhage?**   1 mark

1. Infarction.

❶ A stroke resulting from infarction is visualised as a low-density area (i.e. black on CT scan) with loss of differentiation between grey and white matter. There is often a surrounding whiter area as a result of cerebral oedema. Haemorrhage initially appears as an area of increased density (i.e. white). Occasionally, infarcted brain can become haemorrhagic, causing a further deterioration in the patient's condition.

❶ It is important to differentiate between haemorrhage and infarction (or other pathology) because their management differs. This is not possible clinically and so all patients should have CT of the brain within 48 hours. If the CT scan shows infarction give aspirin (300 mg daily either orally or rectally); this can be started on admission, unless haemorrhage is suspected, and stopped if haemorrhage is shown. Thrombolysis may increasingly be used in the future.

❶ Urgent CT of the brain is indicated with deteriorating consciousness or known coagulopathy to exclude potentially reversible causes, e.g. expanding cerebellar or cerebral haematoma requiring surgical evacuation.

Q **What cerebral artery is affected?**   2 marks

1. Right middle cerebral artery.

❶ The middle cerebral artery supplies the lateral surfaces of the cerebral hemispheres and the optic radiation (cortical branches), as well as the internal capsule (which contains ascending sensory and descending motor tracts). A lesion to the middle cerebral artery may cause weakness and/or sensory loss in the contralateral arm and face (and involvement of the leg if the internal capsule is involved), contralateral homonymous hemianopia, and dysphasia (if dominant hemisphere) or dyspraxia (if non-dominant hemisphere).

❶ A lesion to the anterior cerebral artery, which supplies the medial surfaces of the cerebral hemispheres, may cause motor and/or sensory loss in the contralateral leg.

❶ Lacunar infarcts refer to lesions to the small perforating arteries, arising from the middle and posterior cerebral arteries, which supply the internal capsule, basal ganglia and thalamus. These cause pure motor, sensorimotor or pure sensory stroke with no involvement of higher cortical functions, e.g. no dysphasia.

Q **List six additional investigations that you might consider, briefly explaining why**   3 marks

1. **Full blood count (FBC): excludes polycythaemia and thrombocytosis (increased risk of thrombosis).**

2. **Urea and electrolytes (U&Es): renal impairment may be a result of hypertension.**

3. **Erythrocyte sedimentation rate (ESR): excludes temporal arteritis.**

4. **International normalised ratio (INR): may indicate increased risk of haemorrhage, e.g. if on warfarin.**

5. **Glucose and lipids: secondary prevention of atherosclerosis.**

6. **ECG: for example, excludes AF.**

7. **Echocardiogram: exclude cardiac sources of emboli (see above).**

8. **Carotid Doppler: see below.**

9. **Chest radiograph: for example, excludes lung cancer that causes brain metastases (differential diagnosis).**

205

❶ The above represents a comprehensive list of investigations. Initially, the following tests should be performed: FBC, U&Es, INR, ESR, glucose, lipids, ECG and brain CT scan, with additional investigations where appropriate. In younger patients you may also consider thrombophilia screen and autoantibodies to exclude vasculitis, e.g. systemic lupus erythematosus (SLE – increased risk of thrombosis).

❶ Carotid Doppler is used to exclude internal carotid artery stenosis in surgically fit patients which, depending upon the extent of occlusion (≥ 70 per cent stenosis), can be treated by carotid endarterectomy.

George is transferred to the stroke ward for rehabilitation, where over the following weeks he makes good progress.

Q Name six health professionals involved in George's rehabilitation   **3 marks**

❶ Rehabilitation of stroke patients (in hospital and back in the community) involves a multidisciplinary approach:

1. **Physician/GP: to treat modifiable risk factors such as hypertension, smoking, hyperlipidaemia.**

2. **Dietitian: to address any nutritional problems as a result of the stroke, e.g. dysphagia.**

3. **Physiotherapist: to help reduce spasticity and increase mobility.**

4. **Occupational therapist: to reduce functional disabilities.**

5. **Speech and language therapist: to treat any dysphagia, dysphasia or dysarthria.**

6. **Community nurse: to enable the patient to continue to live at home.**

7. **Social worker: to ensure that the appropriate care package is in place.**

❶ Initially blood pressure after a stroke may be high as a result of disturbance of cerebral autoregulation. It should not be treated in the acute phase because it may impair cerebral perfusion (unless there is coexisting hypertensive encephalopathy).

Total   **20 marks**

NEUROLOGY CASE 2

Ethel, an 82-year-old widow, is admitted after her carer found her that morning still in bed and more confused than normal.

Q List five causes of acute confusion (delirium)   5 marks

1. Infection: in particular urinary tract infection (UTI) and pneumonia and, rarely, meningitis and encephalitis.

2. Metabolic: hypoglycaemia, renal failure, liver failure and electrolyte imbalance, e.g. hyponatraemia.

3. Drugs (and drug withdrawal), e.g. benzodiazepines, opiates, alcohol.

4. Hypoxia: respiratory or cardiac failure.

5. Myocardial infarction.

6. Intracranial lesion, e.g. raised intracranial pressure (ICP), head injury (e.g. subdural haematoma), epilepsy, stroke.

7. Nutritional deficiency: vitamin B_{12}, thiamine (vitamin B_1).

On examination she has a GCS of 11/15, temperature 38.5°C, BP 116/64 mmHg, HR 90 regular, respiratory rate 28/min and pulse oximetry 87 per cent, and there is bronchial breathing at her right lung base.

Q List three non-invasive investigations that you would do   3 marks

1. Chest radiograph: to exclude pneumonia, pulmonary oedema.

2. ECG: exclude myocardial infarction, AF (causing a stroke).

3. Urine dipstick: exclude UTI. Nitrites and leukocytes suggest UTI; if present send a sample for microscopy, culture and sensitivities.

? QUESTIONS
PAGES
46–48

Ethel's blood test results are shown in the table.

Variable	Value	Normal range	Variable	Value	Normal range	Variable	Value	Normal range
Hb (g/dL)	14.8	11.5–16	Sodium (mmol/L)	151	135–145	pH	7.41	7.35–7.45
MCV (fL)	84	76–96	Potassium (mmol/L)	4.1	3.5–5	PO_2 (kPa)	7.6	> 10.6
WCC (neutrophilia) ($\times 10^9$/L)	18	4–11	Urea (mmol/L)	16	2.5–6.7	PCO_2 (kPa)	5.1	4.7–6
Platelets ($\times 10^9$/L)	331	150–400	Creatinine (µmol/L)	211	70–120	HCO_3^- (mmol/L)	24	22–28
CRP (mg/L)	143	< 10	Albumin (g/L)	24	35–50	BE (mmol/L)	–1.2	±2
Glucose (mmol/L)	22.7	4–6	Calcium (mmol/L)	1.93				
			Adjusted calcium	N/A	2.12–2.65			

Q Calculate Ethel's adjusted calcium   1 mark

1. 2.33 mmol/L.

❶ Approximately 50 per cent of plasma calcium is ionised and physiologically important; the remainder is bound to albumin. Ionised calcium is very difficult to measure. However, total plasma calcium can be estimated by adding (or subtracting) 0.1 mmol to calcium concentration for every 4 g/L that albumin is below (or above) 40 g/L. In Ethel's case her albumin level is 24 g/L; subtraction from 40 gives 16; divided by 4 = 4; times 0.1 = 0.4; added to 1.93 = adjusted calcium of 2.33 mmol/L.

❶ Hypoalbuminaemia causes oedema due to reduced intravascular oncotic pressure. Causes include liver failure, nephrotic syndrome, protein-losing enteropathy, malabsorption, malnutrition and malignancy. It is also an acute phase response in infection (levels fall).

Q List five diagnoses inferred from these blood results   5 marks

1. **Type 1 respiratory failure: decreased P_{O_2} (< 8 kPa) with normal P_{CO_2}.**

2. **Dehydration: indicated by increased sodium; also get disproportionately high urea (compared with creatinine).**

3. **Renal impairment: raised urea and creatinine. Although not possible to determine whether this is acute or chronic renal failure, the absence of normocytic anaemia and hypocalcaemia suggests acute renal failure.**

4. **Underlying infection: raised CRP and WCC; neutrophilia suggests bacterial infection.**

5. **Hyperglycaemia: raised glucose.**

❶ In Ethel's case the underlying cause of these abnormal blood results (and her acute confusion) is pneumonia (as indicated by raised CRP/WCC and consolidation on chest examination, later confirmed on chest radiograph) causing type I respiratory failure, dehydration causing hypernatraemia and acute renal failure, and transitory hyperglycaemia (even in the absence of underlying diabetes).

A diagnosis of pneumonia is made and Ethel is successfully treated with oxygen therapy, intravenous antibiotics, sliding scale insulin and intravenous fluids. Before discharge her underlying dementia is assessed and she records an MMSE score of 18.

Q **What MMSE score supports a diagnosis of dementia?**　　　　1 mark

1. **MMSE < 25 supports a diagnosis of dementia.**

❶ MMSE is scored out of 30: 28–30 does not support a diagnosis of dementia; 25–27 is borderline; < 25 supports a diagnosis of dementia (chronic confusion) in the absence of acute confusion and depression.

Q **What are the two most common causes of dementia?**　　　　1 mark

1. **Alzheimer's disease.**

2. **Vascular/multi-infarct dementia: usually the cumulative effect of many strokes or less commonly one major stroke.**

Neurology

❶ Dementia also occurs in several diseases including Parkinson's disease, Huntington's disease, Creutzfeldt–Jakob disease (CJD) and HIV infection.

Q List four blood tests that you would do to exclude treatable causes of dementia   **4 marks**

1. **Thyroid function tests (TFTs).**

2. **Syphilis serology.**

3. **Liver function tests (LFTs): alcohol abuse causes raised γ-glutamyl transferase (GGT).**

4. **FBC: macrocytic anaemia may suggest vitamin B$_{12}$ or folate deficiency; macrocytosis without anaemia is a marker of alcohol abuse.**

5. **Vitamin B$_{12}$, thiamine (vitamin B$_1$) and folate levels.**

❶ Treatable causes of dementia include hypothyroidism, tertiary syphilis, vitamin B$_{12}$, thiamine (vitamin B$_1$) and folate deficiency, chronic alcohol abuse (e.g. cerebral atrophy, Wernicke–Korsakoff syndrome), brain tumours and subdural haematoma.

❶ Dementia is diagnosed clinically but secondary causes must be excluded because some causes are potentially reversible; investigations should include the above blood tests and CT of the brain (to confirm presence of cerebral atrophy and exclude other lesions, e.g. subdural haematoma).

Total   **20 marks**

NEUROLOGY CASE 3

Matthew, an 18-year-old student, is found by his flatmates complaining of headache, stiff neck and photophobia. Worried that he may have meningitis, they rush him straight to A&E.

Q **Name two signs associated with meningeal irritation**   2 marks

1. **Kernig's sign: on lying supine with the knees and hips flexed, there is back pain on extending the knees.**

2. **Brudzinski's sign: on lying supine, flexion of the neck causes flexion of the hips and knees.**

❶ If positive these signs confirm irritation of the meninges, which occurs in meningitis. Similarly, flexing the neck to assess any resistance to movement or associated pain also suggests meningeal irritation (although local infections and arthritis of the spine may also cause neck stiffness).

Before an LP is performed Matthew is examined to exclude raised ICP.

Q **List six signs suggesting raised ICP**   6 marks

1. **Drowsiness, confusion, decreased consciousness.**

2. **Severe headache.**

3. **Irritability.**

4. **Seizures.**

5. **Vomiting.**

6. **False localising signs, e.g. cranial nerve III and VI palsies.**

7. **Irregular respiration, e.g. Cheyne–Stokes respiration (alternating hyperventilation and apnoea).**

QUESTIONS
PAGES
49–51

Neurology

8. **Bradycardia and raised BP (Cushing's response – this is a late sign).**

9. **Papilloedema (late sign) or absence of venous pulsation at the optic disc.**

10. **Opisthotonus, i.e. arching of back and neck (late sign).**

ⓘ Raised ICP can cause tentorial herniation i.e. herniation of the cerebral hemispheres through the tentorial hiatus of the cerebellar tentorium, causing compression of the mid-brain (this may also cause coning of the brain stem through the foramen magnum). If this happens it may cause decreased conscious level (as a result of compression of reticular formation in the brain stem), cardiorespiratory depression (caused by compression of the medulla), and false localising signs, e.g. cranial nerve III and VI palsies (resulting from the long pathways of these cranial nerves).

Q Give two contraindications (other than raised ICP) to LP   **2 marks**

1. **Impaired clotting, e.g. warfarin: may cause a haematoma, resulting in spinal cord compression.**

2. **Thrombocytopenia (platelet count $< 40 \times 10^9$/L): as above.**

3. **Local infection near the site of the puncture: may introduce infection into the CSF.**

4. **Cardiorespiratory instability.**

ⓘ LP is diagnostic in meningitis. However, it is carried out only if there are no signs of raised ICP (otherwise need to perform a CT brain scan to exclude raised ICP). This is because raised cranial pressure may cause coning of the brain stem if CSF pressure below this level is reduced by an LP.

ⓘ Treatment should not be delayed while awaiting an LP (or pending results). If meningitis is suspected but the organism is unknown, give high-dose intravenous cephalosporin, e.g. cefotaxime 2 g, and intravenous dexamethasone (reduces the frequency of complications, *particularly if pneumococcal meningitis is suspected – see below*).

There are no signs of raised ICP and an LP is performed.

Q Indicate (↑, → or ↓) where marked '?' for the expected CSF changes in bacterial meningitis   **3 marks**

	Normal	Bacterial meningitis	TB	Viral meningitis
Appearance	Clear	Turbid	Turbid	Clear
WCC (/mm³)	5 (no neutrophils)	↑↑(200–300) (neutrophils)	Lymphocytes	Lymphocytes
Protein (g/L)	0.2–0.4	↑ (> 1.5)	1–5	< 1.0
Glucose (% plasma glucose)	> 50	↓ (< 50)	< 50	> 50

❶ Other tests performed include: FBC, U&Es, LFTs, CRP, coagulation screen, plasma glucose (to compare with CSF), culture of blood and throat swabs for bacteria (preferably before antibiotics), rapid antigen test for meningitis organisms (on blood, urine and/or CSF).

Matthew is diagnosed with meningococcal meningitis, his CSF Gram stain confirming Neisseria meningitidis.

Q What colour does *Neisseria meningitidis* Gram stain?   **1 mark**

1. **Pink: *N. meningitidis* is a Gram-negative diplococcus.**

❶ Causative organisms of bacterial meningitis vary with the patient's age. In neonates the most common are: *E. coli, Listeria monocytogenes* and β-haemolytic streptococci. In children: *Haemophilus influenzae* (unless immunised), *Streptococcus pneumoniae* and *N. meningitidis* (meningococcal). In teenagers and adults: *N. meningitides* and *S. pneumoniae.* TB causes a subacute onset of meningeal symptoms.

❶ Viral causes of meningitis include mumps, herpes simplex virus (HSV), HIV and Epstein–Barr virus (EBV). Non-infective meningeal inflammation can also be caused by malignant infiltration (e.g. leukaemia), sarcoidosis and SLE.

Neurology

❶ Encephalitis is inflammation of the brain parenchyma (causing focal CNS or psychiatric features, e.g. odd behaviours), although there will also be some degree of accompanying meningeal inflammation (causing meningitis features). CT often shows diffuse areas of oedema typically affecting the temporal lobes; CSF shows lymphocytosis with normal protein and glucose and polymerase chain reaction (PCR) performed for HSV. All patients should be given intravenous aciclovir (10 mg/kg three times daily for 10 days) to treat potential HSV encephalitis.

Q **List four complications of bacterial meningitis**　　　　**4 marks**

1. **Death: untreated acute bacterial meningitis is almost always fatal.**

2. **Learning disability (mental handicap).**

3. **Sensorineural deafness.**

4. **Focal neurological lesions, e.g. cranial nerve palsies.**

5. **Epilepsy.**

6. **Hydrocephalus: as a result of impaired resorption of CSF and may require a ventricular shunt.**

❶ In meningococcal infection septicaemia may predominate, causing septic shock, e.g. delayed capillary refill time (> 2 seconds), and a petechial rash with or without meningitis features. Such patients may deteriorate rapidly with disseminated intravascular coagulation and multiorgan failure; they require high-dose empirical intravenous cephalosporins, aggressive fluid resuscitation and transfer to an intensive care unit.

Q **What prophylaxis do you give to contacts of Matthew and what do you warn them about?**　　　　**2 marks**

1. **Rifampicin (600 mg twice daily for 2 days).**

2. **Warn them about pink-coloured tears and urine.**

Total　　　　**20 marks**

Neurology

OBSTETRICS AND GYNAECOLOGY CASES: ANSWERS

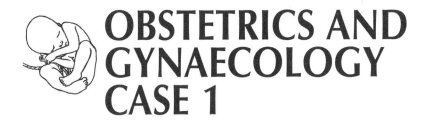

OBSTETRICS AND GYNAECOLOGY CASE 1

Katie, who is 28 weeks into her first pregnancy, suddenly experiences a gush of fluid vaginally in the absence of any uterine contractions. CTG is normal and ultrasonography shows reduced residual amniotic fluid. A speculum examination is performed, which reveals a closed cervix and pooling of fluid in the posterior vaginal fornix.

Q **List four causes of preterm prelabour rupture of membranes (PPROM)** 2 marks

1. **Chorioamnionitis: infection of placental tissues and amniotic fluid.**

2. **Cervical incompetence.**

3. **Antepartum haemorrhage (in particular placental abruption).**

4. **Urinary tract infection (UTI).**

5. **Multiple gestation.**

6. **Polyhydramnios.**

❶ The main causes of PPROM are infection and cervical incompetence. The main risks after PPROM are maternal/neonatal infection, fetal distress and a prolapsed cord.

❶ A nitrazine stick can be used to detect the presence of amniotic fluid (to confirm PPROM) in the vagina (goes black).

Q **From what common vaginal organism is Katie's baby at risk?** 1 mark

1. **Group B streptococcus (GBS).**

QUESTIONS PAGES 55–58

❶ Group B streptococcus is a common organism, present in the vagina of up to 25 per cent of women. It may very rarely infect the neonate, either during delivery or via ascending infection (e.g. after PPROM) and cause pneumonia, septicaemia or meningitis. In the UK (in contrast to the USA) pregnant women are not routinely screened for GBS unless there are risk factors present (e.g. pre-term labour, pre-term rupture of membranes, previous GBS infection, fever during labour). Current guidelines recommend the use of antibiotics (penicillin or clindamycin) during labour only and not prophylactically in the antenatal period.

Q List two treatments to decrease perinatal complications   2 marks

❶ In most cases PPROM is followed by onset of premature labour. In those cases that do not, the dilemma is balancing the advantages of continuing pregnancy (so as to increase fetal maturity) against the risk of chorioamnionitis (which may cause perinatal death). The risks can be reduced by:

1. **Intramuscular betamethasone: should be given to all mothers < 34 weeks to promote fetal lung maturity and reduce the risk of respiratory distress syndrome (RDS). Two doses are given, 12–24 h apart.**

2. **Intravenous antibiotics, e.g. benzylpenicillin, during labour.**

❶ Tocolytics (e.g. nifedipine, given to suppress contractions) should be considered only in women who require transfer to a tertiary centre or to allow some time for antenatal corticosteroids to be administered.

On examination Katie's temperature is 38°C, heart rate 92 beats/min and she has raised inflammatory markers. As a result of the risks of maternal and fetal infection it is decided to induce labour. Her cervix is assessed using Bishop's score.

Q List four features used to assess Bishop's score   2 marks

Feature	Bishop's score			
	0	1	2	3
Dilatation (cm)	< 1	1–2	2–4	> 4
Length of cervix (cm)	> 4	2–4	1–2	< 1
Station (relative to ischial spines)	−3	−2	−1/0	+1/+2
Consistency	Firm	Medium	Soft	Soft
Position	Posterior	Middle	Anterior	Anterior

Q **What Bishop's score (BS) is considered ripe for induction?** 1 mark

1. **A BS > 5 indicates that the cervix is favourable for induction.**

ℹ If nulliparous women are induced with an unripe cervix, the risks of prolonged labour, fetal distress and caesarean section are increased.

Q **What is used to make the cervix ripe for induction?** 1 mark

1. **Intravaginal prostaglandin pessary (or gel).**

ℹ Most inductions are started with prostaglandins. Once the cervix is ripe artificial rupture of the membranes (ARM) is performed (not relevant in this case); oxytocin infusion may be used to augment contractions.

Katie's contractions are inefficient so she is started with an infusion of oxytocin.

Q **List two potential complications of using oxytocin in Katie** 2 marks

1. **Uterine hyperstimulation: uterus should contract ≤ 4/10 min. Excessive contractions may cause fetal distress. When labour is induced the fetus requires regular/continuous CTG monitoring.**

2. **Water intoxication: oxytocin has antidiuretic hormone (ADH)-like effects. The risk is reduced by restricting infusion volume.**

ℹ In multiparous women oxytocin may also cause uterine rupture.

Obstetrics

❶ When augmenting labour, it should be used with care because delay may be a result of cephalopelvic disproportion (CPD) as opposed to inefficient uterine contractions.

Katie delivers a girl called Emma weighing 1.1 kg. At 1 min of life Emma's extremities are bluish, her limbs flaccid, her breathing irregular, she grimaces when the soles of her feet are stimulated and her heart rate is 82 beats/min.

Q Calculate Emma's 1-minute Apgar score　　　　　　　　**2 marks**

1. Apgar score of 4.

Apgar score	0	1	2
Colour	White/blue	**Extremities blue, body pink**	Pink
Heart rate	Absent	**< 100**	> 100
Respiratory effort	Absent	**Gasping or irregular**	Regular strong cry
Muscle tone	**Flaccid**	Some flexion of limbs	Active movement
Reflex irritability	Absent	**Grimace**	Cry

Within an hour of birth Emma starts developing signs of respiratory distress. She is intubated by the neonatologist, artificial surfactant is instilled and she is artificially ventilated.

Q List four pulmonary causes of respiratory distress in a neonate　　**2 marks**

1. Transient tachypnoea of the newborn: caused by delay in resorption of lung fluid.

2. Respiratory distress syndrome (RDS): caused by insufficient surfactant production. Affects majority of neonates born before or at 28 weeks.

3. Meconium aspiration.

4. Pneumonia, e.g. group B streptococcal infection is a common cause of neonatal pneumonia (increased risk with PPROM).

5. Pneumothorax: spontaneously occurs in up to 1 per cent of deliveries,

Obstetrics

although often asymptomatic.

6. Milk aspiration, e.g. as a result of a tracheo-oesophageal fistula, gastro-oesophageal reflux or cleft palate.

7. Persistent pulmonary hypertension of the newborn: results from high pulmonary vascular resistance causing right-to-left shunting of blood flow within the heart.

ⓘ Non-pulmonary causes include congenital heart disease, birth asphyxia and severe anaemia.

Q List two complications from artificially ventilating Emma   2 marks

1. Retinopathy of prematurity: immature retinal vessels are sensitive to fluctuations in Pao_2, causing vascular proliferation and leading to retinal detachment and blindness.

2. Pulmonary interstitial emphysema (PIE): as a result of air from overinflated alveoli tracking into the interstitium, reduces lung compliance and worsens respiratory failure.

3. Pneumothorax.

4. Chronic lung disease of prematurity (bronchopulmonary dysplasia): defined as O_2 requirements after 36 weeks' gestational age. Ventilation causes lung damage from pressure trauma, O_2 toxicity and infection.

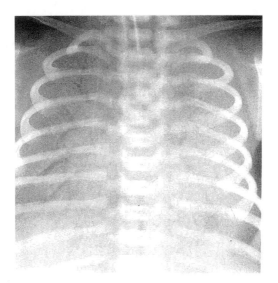

221

Emma's chest radiograph is shown.

Q **Describe three abnormalities on the chest radiograph**   3 marks

1. **Endotracheal tube (lies at appropriate position at the level of the clavicles).**

2. **Air bronchograms (air in the airways surrounded by solid lung).**

3. **Widespread (or diffuse) shadowing (opacification) of the lungs, often described as ground-glass appearance.**

4. **Indistinct or obscured heart border.**

❶ These chest radiograph changes are characteristic of RDS.

Total   **20 marks**

REFERENCES

❶ The following Royal College of Obstetricians and Gynaecologists guidelines are freely available at www.rcog.org.uk

Induction of Labour. **Guideline no. 9. June 2001.**

Prevention of Early Onset Neonatal Group B Streptococcal Disease. **Guideline no. 36. November 2003**

Antenatal Corticosteroids to Prevent Respiratory Distress Syndrome. **Guideline no. 7. February 2004.**

Preterm Prelabour Rupture of Membranes. **Guideline no. 44. November 2006.**

Obstetrics

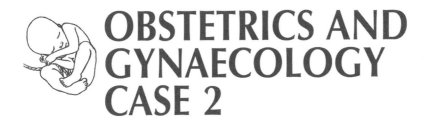# OBSTETRICS AND GYNAECOLOGY CASE 2

Paul and Julie (both aged 33 years) visit their GP after 2 years of being unable to conceive. A full history is taken from both. Julie's gynaecological history reveals irregular periods.

Q What general advice would you give to couples trying to get pregnant   2 marks

1. **Timing of intercourse: recommend intercourse every 2–3 days. It is not recommended to attempt to time intercourse around ovulation because this is unreliable and stressful.**

2. **Stop smoking: smoking is associated with decreased fertility in women and reduced semen quality in men.**

3. **Reduce alcohol intake: excessive alcohol intake in women carries risks for the fetus (fetal alcohol syndrome); in men excessive alcohol intake reduces semen quality.**

4. **Optimise weight: a body mass index (BMI) < 19 (with irregular periods) or > 29 is likely to be associated with reduced female fertility. In addition men with a BMI > 29 are likely to have reduced fertility.**

5. **Several occupations are associated with reduced fertility, e.g. those in close contact with agents such as chemicals, heat and radiation (anaesthetists, laboratory workers, agricultural workers, bakers and radiotherapists)**

6. **Pre-conception advice, e.g. rubella screening, folic acid 0.4 mg.**

❶ Eighty-four per cent of couples in the general population will have conceived within 1 year of having regular unprotected sexual intercourse; 50 per cent of women who do not conceive in the first year are likely to do so in the second year.

QUESTIONS PAGES 59–61

🛈 Infertility is defined as the inability to conceive after 2 years of regular unprotected intercourse in the absence of reproductive pathology.

Q **List four points in the full history suggestive of tubal dysfunction**   **4 marks**

1. **Abdominal or pelvic surgery, e.g. appendectomy.**

2. **Endometriosis.**

3. **Peritonitis, e.g. as a complication of appendicitis.**

4. **History of pelvic inflammatory disease (PID) or a sexually transmitted infection (STI).**

5. **Previous ectopic pregnancy.**

6. **Tubal ligation (for sterilisation).**

🛈 It is estimated that tubal factors are responsible for approximately 14 per cent of infertility cases. Tubal disease includes pelvic adhesions and tubal obstruction:

- Pelvic adhesions (1–3): may affect tubal motility and ovum pick-up. Laparoscopy is the investigation of choice to assess the pelvis, tubes and ovaries.

- Tubal obstruction (4–6): impaired tubal patency is investigated by a dye test during laparoscopic hysterosalpingography (radio-opaque dye is instilled through the cervix and should 'leak out' at the end of the tubes) or by hysterosalpingo-contrast sonography).

As an initial assessment the GP organises a semen analysis for Paul and requests a number of blood tests for Julie.

Q List three variables measured in semen analysis   **3 marks**

Variable	Normal range
Volume	> 2 ml
Liquefaction time	Within 60 min
Sperm concentration	> 20 × 10⁶/ml
Total sperm count	> 40 × 10⁶
Motility	> 50% with normal progression
Morphology	> 30% with normal morphology
White cell count	< 1 × 10⁶/ml.

ℹ If the initial analysis is abnormal another semen specimen is evaluated before diagnosis is made. The best time for the second sample is at least 3 months after the initial sample because the cycle of spermatozoa formation takes about 3 months to complete. In the UK, a low sperm count or quality is found to be the only cause of infertility in about 20 per cent of couples and is a contributory factor in a further 25 per cent of couples.

The results come back confirming normal semen analysis. Her blood results are shown in the table.

LH (day 2) (U/L)	18 (normal range 3–16)
FSH (day 2) (U/L)	6 (normal range 2–8)
Progesterone (day 21 – mid-luteal) (nmol/L)	8

Q What is a normal day 21 progesterone concentration?   **1 mark**

1. > 25 nmol/L.

❶ The progesterone level is the most commonly used test to assess whether ovulation occurs. Ovulation refers to the release of an egg from the mature follicle in the ovary, stimulated by an LH surge. The mature follicle forms the corpus luteum, which under the influence of LH secretes progesterone; this prepares the endometrium for implantation. In the absence of pregnancy, progesterone levels begin to decline about 7 days after ovulation and this results in shedding of the endometrial lining (menstruation). In a 28-day cycle ovulation occurs 2 weeks before the next period and progesterone levels peak on day 21 (mid-luteal phase).

Q **Give two explanations for Julie's progesterone concentration**   2 marks

1. **Anovulation, e.g. as a result of polycystic ovarian syndrome.**

2. **Incorrect cycle dates.**

❶ Irregular periods cause difficulty in calculating when ovulation occurs and therefore on what day to measure progesterone levels. Under such circumstances measure 7 days before the next suspected period, although this may need to be repeated if dates are subsequently incorrect.

Q **What might an FSH much greater than 10 U/L on day 2 suggest?**   1 mark

1. **Premature menopause.**

❶ Advanced female age is associated with follicular decline and malfunction. Over time the follicles become resistant to gonadotrophin stimulation and, coupled with a decreased negative feedback from oestrogens, this leads to an increase in FSH and LH. This indicates primary ovarian failure causing premature menopause (in someone who is 33). In the UK the average age for menopause is 51 years.

Q **What is your likely diagnosis?**   1 mark

1. **Polycystic ovarian syndrome (PCOS).**

❶ PCOS is associated with irregular cycles, anovulation, raised LH producing an LH:FSH ratio ≥ 2:1 (normally 1:1) and androgen excess. Ultrasonography can demonstrate polycystic ovaries ('string of pearls' sign, i.e. peripheral small cysts [follicles] > 12 with increased ovarian volume).

Q List three clinical features that Julie might have 3 marks

❶ Typical clinical features of PCOS are:

1. **Obesity: approximately 40 per cent of women with PCOS are obese.**

2. **Acne.**

3. **Virilisation: development of male secondary sexual characteristics, e.g. deep voice, clitoromegaly.**

4. **Hirsutism: presence of excessive facial and bodily hair in a male pattern (although may be disguised).**

5. **Menstrual disturbance: amenorrhoea, oligomenorrhoea, dysfunctional uterine bleeding (irregular or excessive uterine bleeding in the absence of a cause).**

❶ PCOS is related to hyperinsulinaemia and insulin resistance causing excessive androgen secretion. Obesity worsens the underlying androgen excess as a result of adipose tissue conversion of oestrogens to androgens. Treatment of infertility involves weight loss and ovulation induction with clomifene. Metformin is being increasingly used although it is not yet licensed for the treatment of PCOS.

Julie is referred to her local infertility clinic. She has a hysterosalpingogram which is normal. Her infertility is treated with clomifene.

Q List three complications associated with this treatment 3 marks

1. **Ovarian hyperstimulation syndrome (OHSS): OHSS causes abdominal distension as a result of ovarian enlargement and cyst formation. Severe hyperstimulation can cause thromboembolic events, ascites and pulmonary effusions. Prevention requires careful monitoring via ultrasonography and early recognition of the symptoms.**

2. **Multiple pregnancy: affects approximately 20 per cent of clomifene-treated pregnancies.**

3. **Ovarian cancer: may increase risk of ovarian cancer and therefore its use is restricted to 12 months.**

Obstetrics

❶ Ovulatory disorders are responsible for 20 per cent of infertility cases. The cause is unexplained in 30 per cent of couples.

❶ Clomifene is an oestrogen antagonist that acts by preventing normal negative oestrogen feedback in the hypothalamus, thereby increasing gonadotrophin-releasing hormone (GnRH) and hence gonadotrophins that stimulate the ovary to produce more follicles.

Total   **20 marks**

REFERENCES

❶ Available from Royal College of Obstetricians and Gynaecologist: www.rcog.org.uk

Fertility: Assessment and treatment for people with fertility problems. **Guideline no. 11. February 2004.**

Revised 2003 consensus on diagnostic criteria and long-term health risks related to polycystic ovary syndrome. *Fertility and Sterility* **2004;81:19–25.**

Obstetrics

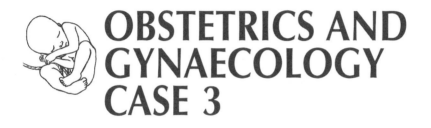

OBSTETRICS AND GYNAECOLOGY CASE 3

Debbie, aged 26 years, is out walking when her waters break. She is rushed to the labour ward by her husband Gerald, complaining of regular painful contractions every 10 minutes.

Q List four questions that you would ask   2 marks

1. **When is the baby due?**

2. **Have you felt the baby move?**

3. **Is it a single pregnancy or twins?**

4. **Are you aware of any problems with the pregnancy, e.g. malpresentation?**

5. **Is the liquor coloured (is there any meconium)?**

6. **Do you have any medical problems, e.g. diabetes?**

7. **Any problems with previous pregnancies including delivery?**

❶ The aim of these questions is to assess any risk to the baby and mother, e.g. is the baby premature? Previous poor pregnancy outcomes are risk factors for this pregnancy; passage of meconium may indicate that the fetus is distressed, but can be normal in a post-term pregnancy.

On obstetric palpation fundal height corresponds to her dates (she is 39 weeks' pregnant with her first child), the lie is longitudinal, the presentation cephalic and the fetal head engaged. On vaginal examination the position is left occipitoanterior and the cervix is 4 cm dilated.

Q List six *maternal* observations recorded on the partogram   3 marks

QUESTIONS
PAGES
62–65

❶ The partogram is a graphic record of labour allowing a visual record of cervical dilatation against the expected norm plus key maternal and fetal observations, thus allowing active management if required:

1. **Heart rate, blood pressure and temperature.**

2. **Strength and frequency of contractions.**

3. **Cervical dilatation.**

4. **Urine volume: to exclude maternal dehydration.**

5. **Urinalysis e.g. proteinuria, ketonuria.**

6. **Intravenous infusions, e.g. oxytocin.**

7. **Any drugs, e.g. pethidine.**

8. **Liquor, i.e. colour of vaginal discharge.**

9. **Station: indicating the descent of the presenting part, in relation to the ischial spines.**

❶ Fetal observations include heart rate (normal range 110–160 beats/min), position (displayed graphically), extent of fixing/engagement, moulding or caput.

Debbie's contractions become progressively more frequent and painful. Three hours later her cervical dilatation is reassessed and plotted on the partogram, demonstrating that Debbie's labour is progressing satisfactorily.

Q Give two examples each of non-pharmacological and pharmacological methods of pain relief   **2 marks**

1. **Non-pharmacological (typically used during latent phase), e.g. transcutaneous electrical nerve stimulation (TENS), back massage, relaxation and breathing exercises, and a warm bath.**

2. **Pharmacological (typically used during active phase and stage 2), e.g. nitric oxide + O_2 (gas and air), pethidine, epidural, morphine.**

Q By how many centimetres should the cervix be dilated by now?   **1 mark**

1. **7 cm, i.e. an increase of 3 cm above last recording 3 hours ago of 4 cm.**

❶ Progress in the active phase (of the first stage of labour) is assessed
by cervical dilatation from 3 cm to fully dilated (10 cm) and effaced.
Dilatation typically proceeds at 1 cm/h in a primigravida and 2 cm/h in a
multigravida.

Q **List four causes of failure to progress in the first stage of labour**   **2 marks**

1. **Inefficient uterine contractions (e.g. as a result of dehydration).**

2. **Malpresentation, e.g. face presentation, breech.**

3. **Malposition, e.g. occiput posterior.**

4. **Cephalopelvic disproportion (CPD): disproportion between the fetal head
and maternal pelvis.**

5. **Cervical dystocia: failure of cervical dilatation (e.g. as a result of previous
trauma, surgery).**

❶ Primary dysfunctional labour is slow progress during the active phase of
labour (usually as a result of inefficient contractions). Secondary arrest
is initial satisfactory progress, followed by arrest after 7 cm dilatation
(usually caused by CPD or malposition). Causes of delay in the second
stage of labour (which should last < 1 h in a primigravida) include CPD
(preventing internal rotation, termed 'deep transverse arrest'), occiput
posterior position, secondary uterine inertia, maternal exhaustion, pain
and anxiety.

*During labour, Debbie's baby is intermittently monitored by CTG to
assess whether her baby is distressed.*

Q **What four components are used to interpret a CTG?**   **2 marks**

❶ CTG monitors fetal heart rate alongside uterine contractions and is used
in labour to detect fetal hypoxia (supported by passage of fresh meconium
and fetal scalp pH < 7.2). The four components used in interpreting a CTG
are:

1. **Baseline heart rate: should be 110–160 beats/min (abnormal if < 100 or
> 180).**

Obstetrics

2. **Baseline variability: baseline heart rate should vary between 6 and 25 beats/min (abnormal if varies < 5 beats/min over a 90-min period).**

3. **Accelerations: defined as increase in heart rate of ≥ 15 beats/min (from the baseline) for ≥ 15 s in response to uterine activity. Reassuring feature.**

4. **Decelerations: defined as decrease in heart rate of ≥ 15 beats/min (from the baseline) for ≥ 15 s. The timing of the deceleration in relation to the contractions classifies them into: early: trough of deceleration coincides with peak of contraction and is usually considered a normal response to the uterine contraction; late: considered abnormal; or variable: interpretation more complex.**

❶ If CTG is abnormal, lie the mother on her left side (to avoid compression of the vena cava, stop any oxytocin infusion and take fetal scalp blood sample. If pH < 7.2 deliver immediately.

Q **List four sequential stages in the passage of the fetus through the birth canal leading up to the delivery of the shoulders**   **4 marks**

1. **Head engages typically in occiput transverse position.**

2. **Head descends further into the pelvis.**

3. **Head flexes onto chest so that the most favourable (smallest) diameter of the fetal skull presents.**

4. **Internal rotation (directed by the gutter-shaped pelvic floor) so that the head arrives at the pelvic outlet in the anteroposterior position.**

5. **Head extends from underneath the pubic symphysis, starting to distend the vulva, allowing the head to be delivered. This is known as crowning.**

6. **Restitution of the head so that it aligns with the obliquely placed shoulders.**

7. **External rotation: the delivered head rotates to lie in the transverse position so that the shoulders lie in an anteroposterior plane.**

❶ This is followed by delivery of the anterior shoulder, followed by the posterior shoulder and finally the rest of the body.

Debbie delivers a pink and healthy boy called Alex who cries immediately.

Obstetrics

Q List four steps in your immediate management of Alex   **2 marks**

1. **Clamp and cut cord.**

2. **Dry baby and wrap in warm towel.**

3. **Record 1-minute Apgar score.**

4. **Rapid inspection for gross abnormalities and birth injuries.**

5. **Give intramuscular vitamin K (if it has been previously discussed and agreed with the mother).**

6. **Attach label for identification.**

7. **Hand to mother for early skin-to-skin contact and suckling.**

As Alex is born, Debbie is given intramuscular Syntometrine (oxytocin with ergometrine). After the birth the placenta is removed by controlled cord traction and inspected for completeness.

Q Give two non-pharmacological techniques for reducing PPH   **1 mark**

❶ Uterine contraction, which is under hormonal control of oxytocin, can be increased by:

1. **Early suckling: stimulates oxytocin release from post-pituitary gland**

2. **Rubbing up a uterine contraction: massage the fundus to stimulate a contraction.**

❶ PPH is bleeding from the genital tract after either vaginal delivery or caesarean section (more common after a caesarean section). Primary PPH is defined as > 500 ml blood loss in the first 24 h after delivery (secondary PPH refers to any blood loss after 24 h post-delivery). It is caused by failure of the uterus to contract (70 per cent), damage to the genital tract (20 per cent), retained tissue, inverted uterus or coagulation disorder. PPH accounts for significant maternal mortality, causing a third of maternal deaths post partum in the developed world.

Q Name two drugs that are used in the management of PPH   **1 mark**

Obstetrics

1. **Oxytocin: as a stat dose or infusion to help the uterus contract.**

2. **Ergometrine: careful in hypertensive patients because it may cause a sudden rise in blood pressure.**

3. **Prostaglandin analogues, e.g. carboprost (given intramuscularly) and misoprostol (given orally, per vagina or per rectum).**

❶ These drugs increase uterine contraction and cause vasoconstriction, thereby preventing the uterus from becoming atonic.

Total   **20 marks**

REFERENCES

❶ Available from Royal College of Obstetricians and Gynaecologists: www.rcog.org.uk

The Use of Electronic Fetal Monitoring. The use and interpretation of cardiotocography in intrapartum fetal surveillance. **Guideline no. 8. May 2001.**

The Management of Postpartum Haemorrhage. **Scottish Obstetric Guidelines and Audit Project. June 1998, update 2002.**

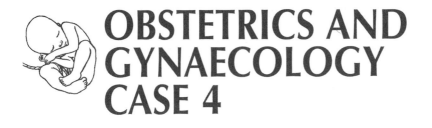

OBSTETRICS AND GYNAECOLOGY
CASE 4

Sue and her husband Peter are both delighted to discover that Sue is pregnant for the first time. Sue is now 10 weeks' pregnant (her LMP was 15 July and her cycle is normally a regular 28 days) and she attends the antenatal clinic for her booking visit.

Q When is Sue's EDD according to Naegele's rule?   1 mark

1. **21 April.**

❶ Naegele's rule states that the due date can be found by taking the first day of a woman's last menstrual period, subtracting 3 months, adding 1 week and adjusting the year if necessary. However, this rule makes the assumption that cycle length is 28 days and is therefore less accurate if ovulation happens early/late or menstrual periods are irregular.

Q List six blood tests that you would offer   3 marks

1. **Full blood count (FBC): to exclude anaemia (< 10.5 g/dl in pregnant women). The most common cause is iron deficiency because iron requirements are increased in pregnancy; it also drops during pregnancy because of haemodilution (as a result of an increase in plasma volume).**

2. **ABO group: in case the mother requires an urgent blood transfusion; also required in investigation of neonatal jaundice (caused by ABO incompatibility between mother and baby).**

3. **Rhesus status.**

QUESTIONS
PAGES
66–69

4. **Rubella antibodies: ideally screen preconception and if negative immunise (measles, mumps, rubella or MMR vaccine) and practice safe sex for ≥ 3 months. If negativity is discovered only at the booking visit, educate on importance of avoiding contact with infected individuals, and immunise postnatally.**

5. **Syphilis serology: need to exclude syphilis that may cause congenital syphilis.**

6. **Hepatitis B virus and HIV: measures need to be taken to prevent vertical transmission.**

❶ Also offer urine dipstick. If a UTI is suspected send sample for culture. Asymptomatic bacteriuria during pregnancy can progress to pyelonephritis, which is associated with pre-term labour, fetal death and IUGR. Proteinuria in conjunction with raised blood pressure may indicate pre-eclampsia (occurs later in pregnancy).

❶ Rhesus haemolytic disease occurs when a rhesus-negative mother gives birth to a rhesus-positive baby. If rhesus-positive fetal cells cross the placenta the mother may produce anti-rhesus antibodies (anti-D are the most common antibodies), which in a subsequent pregnancy may cross the placenta into the fetal circulation and cause haemolysis. To prevent isoimmunisation all rhesus-negative women are given anti-D antibodies at 28 and 34 weeks and after any potential 'leaks', e.g. abortion, ectopic pregnancy, amniocentesis/chorionic villous sampling (CVS) and antepartum haemorrhage.

Q List four examples of dietary advice that you would give Sue   2 marks

1. **Take 400 µg/day folic acid: this should ideally be taken preconception and during the first trimester to reduce risks of neural tube defects (e.g. anencephaly, spina bifida).**

2. **Eat plenty of fruit and vegetables.**

3. **Avoid vitamin A supplementation (potentially teratogenic) and liver (which contains high vitamin A levels).**

4. **Prevent listeria infection (may cause mid-trimester miscarriage, pre-term labour, congenital listeriosis) by avoiding drinking unpasteurised milk, soft cheeses (e.g. brie, paté) and any uncooked/undercooked meats.**

5. Prevent toxoplasmosis infection (may cause congenital abnormalities) by avoiding raw/undercooked meats (e.g. steaks) and always washing hands after handling raw meat.

6. Prevent salmonella infection (may cause neonatal septicaemia) by avoiding raw eggs including mayonnaise and raw/undercooked meats, especially poultry.

7. Avoid alcohol in first trimester (may cause fetal alcohol syndrome) and limit intake to 1 unit/day thereafter.

Q List eight common minor symptoms of pregnancy that Sue may experience   4 marks

1. Nausea and vomiting: affect up to 75 per cent of women. It is typically worse during the first trimester.

2. Backache: common in late pregnancy. Felt over the sacroiliac joints as result of progesterone-mediated relaxation of ligaments and muscles.

3. Breathlessness: caused by progesterone-induced hyperventilation lowering maternal Pa_{CO_2} so as to increase CO_2 exchange across the placenta from fetus to mother.

4. Constipation: caused by progesterone-mediated reduced gut motility, exacerbated in late pregnancy by pressure of enlarged uterus. Ensure adequate fluid and fibre intake.

5. Heartburn: caused by progesterone-mediated relaxation of lower oesophageal sphincter.

6. Headaches, palpitations, fainting: caused by changes in the cardiovascular system (peripheral resistance falls during pregnancy).

7. Urinary frequency: a result of pressure of fetal head on the bladder (need to exclude UTI).

8. Ankle oedema: caused by fluid retention and mechanical obstruction preventing venous return.

9. Carpal tunnel syndrome: as a result of fluid retention.

Obstetrics

10. Itching: common and may be the result of pruritic eruption of pregnancy, i.e. an itchy papular rash. If generalised and severe need to exclude cholestasis of pregnancy (rare condition associated with IUGR and intrauterine death).

As a result of her age Sue has an increased risk of chromosomal abnormalities including Down's syndrome (her risk is 1:338).

Q **Name two markers measured to screen for trisomy 21** 2 marks

1. **Nuchal translucency (NT): ultrasound measurement of translucent subcutaneous space (caused by fluid accumulation) at the back of the fetal neck. Increased thickness of fluid is associated with fetal abnormalities (chromosomal and structural).**

2. **α-Fetoprotein (AFP): low levels of AFP are associated with trisomy 21, high levels are associated with structural abnormalities (e.g. neural tube defects).**

3. **Human chorionic gonadotrophin (hCG): increased in trisomy 21.**

4. **Pregnancy-associated plasma protein A (PAPP-A): decreased in trisomy 21.**

5. **Unconjugated oestriol: decreased in trisomy 21.**

6. **Inhibin A: increased in trisomy 21.**

ⓘ Various combinations of the above are used in the first or second trimester to screen for trisomy 21 (Down's syndrome). For example, in the first trimester (at 10–12 weeks) the combination of NT, hCG and PAPP-A is termed the combined test. These various tests will estimate the risk for a baby of trisomy 21 (based on maternal age). If the risk is high (> 1 in 250), the mother is offered a diagnostic test (e.g. amniocentesis, CVS), although these carry a risk of miscarriage (0.5–2 per cent).

Q **List six symptoms associated with pre-eclampsia** 3 marks

1. **Headaches.**

2. **Visual disturbance, e.g. blurring or flashing.**

3. **Nausea and vomiting.**

4. **Swelling of face, hands and feet.**

238

5. **Epigastric pain.**

6. **Irritability.**

7. **Generalised malaise.**

ⓘ However, pre-eclampsia may also be asymptomatic so regular screening is essential. This involves regular antenatal blood pressure checks and urinalysis for proteinuria. Admit the mother if her blood pressure > 30/20 mmHg above booking BP, or > 160/100 or > 140/90 with proteinuria.

ⓘ Risk factors for pre-eclampsia include: < 20 or > 35 years of age, BMI > 25, nulliparous, previous pre-eclampsia or family history, multiple gestation, and pre-existing hypertension or renal disease (reduced risk in smokers).

Q **What four investigations would you do in pre-eclampsia?**   **2 marks**

1. **Monitor blood pressure.**

2. **Fluid balance/urine output.**

3. **Daily weight measurements.**

4. **Urine dipstick for proteinuria: if positive send off for the protein:creatinine ratio or to measure 24-hour proteinuria**

5. **Bloods: U&Es (renal failure is a late sign), raised urate (early sign), liver function tests (LFTs; deranged), FBC (thrombocytopenia, anaemia), clotting (deranged).**

6. **Fetal monitoring: ultrasonography (for IUGR), CTG.**

ⓘ Pre-eclampsia typically develops after 20 weeks (and usually resolves 10 days after delivery) and is a multisystem disorder affecting the placenta (causing IUGR), kidneys, brain (causing eclampsia), liver, blood (causing haemolysis) and coagulation (causing disseminated intravascular coagulation or DIC). The underlying pathology is poor trophoblastic invasion of the spiral arteries, leading to decreased blood supply to the fetoplacental unit. The maternal cardiovascular response to this is to raise the BP. There is no cure except to terminate the pregnancy and deliver the baby (although in asymptomatic pre-eclampsia BP may be reduced while awaiting fetal maturation).

Obstetrics

239

❶ HELLP syndrome is a very severe form of pre-eclampsia: **h**aemolysis, **e**levated **l**iver enzymes, **l**ow **p**latelet count.

At 28 weeks Sue attends the antenatal clinic for her regular antenatal care. On obstetric examination the midwife finds that the fundal height is 24 cm.

Q Give four reasons why Sue may be small for dates   **2 marks**

1. Incorrect dates.

2. IUGR.

3. Constitutionally small baby.

4. Oligohydramnios, i.e. reduced amniotic fluid.

❶ Fundal height (measured from the fundus to the top of the symphysis pubis in centimetres) gives a rough estimation of the gestational age of the baby in weeks, e.g. at 28 weeks the fundal height should be 28 ± 3 cm.

Q List six causes of IUGR   **3 marks**

❶ Causes of IUGR can be classified as:

1. Maternal causes, e.g. malnutrition, smoking, systemic disease (such as renal disease, anaemia).

2. Placental insufficiency, e.g. multiple gestation, antepartum haemorrhage, anti-phospholipid syndrome (reduces uteroplacental perfusion), inadequate trophoblastic invasion as seen in pre-eclampsia.

3. Fetal causes, e.g. infections (e.g. cytomegalovirus), congenital malformations, chromosomal abnormalities (e.g. Down's syndrome, Turner syndrome)

❶ IUGR can be divided further into symmetrical and asymmetrical forms. Asymmetrical IUGR is caused by placental insufficiency, i.e. the fetus is starved; brain growth (and hence head circumference) is relatively spared at the expense of liver glycogen and fat stores (causing reduced abdominal circumference). Pregnancies at risk of IUGR (e.g. small for dates) can be monitored and a decision made whether to continue the pregnancy or

Obstetrics

deliver the baby on the basis of fetal monitoring, growth charts, gestational age and umbilical artery blood flow (absent or reverse end-diastolic blood flow indicates poor perfusion causing fetal hypoxia).

❶ Babies with IUGR have an increased risk of: hypoxia and death (*in utero* and during labour); hypothermia, hypoglycaemia and jaundice as a result of polycythaemia (postnatally); and type 2 diabetes, hypertension and cardiovascular disease (in adulthood).

Q List six topics that you want to discuss with Sue in her third trimester 3 marks

1. **Signs of labour: painful contractions occurring at less than 10-minute intervals, show (blood/mucus plug) and rupture of amniotic membranes.**

2. **Birth plan, e.g. where does she want to have the baby – home or hospital?**

3. **Pain management during delivery, e.g. epidural, gas and air.**

4. **How does she intend to feed the baby? Outline the benefits of breast-feeding.**

5. **Local antenatal classes: to prepare for delivery and preparation for the postnatal period.**

6. **Future contraceptive plans, e.g. cannot use COC if breast-feeding.**

Total **25 marks**

REFERENCES

❶ Available from Royal College of Obstetricians and Gynaecologists: www.rcog.org.uk

Antenatal Screening for Down's Syndrome. July 2003.

Antenatal Care: Routine care for the healthy pregnant woman. Guideline no. 6. October 2003.

Obstetrics

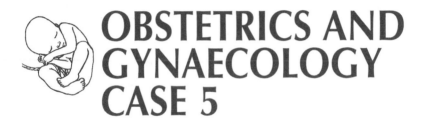

OBSTETRICS AND GYNAECOLOGY CASE 5

Ageeth, a 26-year-old woman, visits her GP on Monday requesting emergency contraception. She recently started a new relationship and had unprotected sexual intercourse on Saturday night. She is on day 9 of her 28-day cycle.

Q **What would you advise Ageeth?** 2 marks

1. **She is at risk of pregnancy and should be offered emergency contraception (EC).**

2. **She could have hormonal EC (levonorgestrel) within 72 h of unprotected sexual intercourse (UPSI); the sooner she takes this the more effective it is.**

3. **She could have a copper IUD (intrauterine device) fitted. This is more effective than hormonal EC and she could use it for future contraception as well. This can be fitted up to 5 days after UPSI or up to 5 days after earliest expected date of ovulation (whichever is the latest). In this example, she has a 28-day cycle, so the copper IUD could be fitted up until day 19 of her cycle. This is because implantation happens at least 5 days after ovulation.**

She opts for hormonal emergency contraception and chooses the pill for future contraception.

Q **Describe two contraceptive mechanisms of COCs** 2 marks

1. **Oestrogen and progesterone exert negative feedback on GnRH, LH and FSH, preventing follicular development and ovulation.**

2. **Progestogen causes endometrial atrophy, preventing implantation.**

QUESTIONS
PAGES
70–73

3. Progestogen acts on cervical mucus, making it hostile to ascending sperm.

❶ The COC contains both oestrogen and progestogen. In general the preparation with the lowest content of both to provide good cycle control is prescribed (to minimise side effects). The COC is one of the most reliable and popular methods of contraception and, if used properly, fewer than 1 in 100 women will become pregnant in a year.

Q **List eight *absolute* contraindications to the COC**   4 marks

1. **Pregnancy (although there is no evidence that the COC harms the fetus).**

2. **Breast-feeding < 6 weeks post partum.**

3. **Ischaemic heart disease (IHD) or multiple risk factors for IHD, e.g. diabetes, hypertensive, family history.**

4. **Smoker: aged ≥ 35 years and smoking > 15 cigarettes a day.**

5. **Obesity: BMI > 40 kg/m² (as increased risk of IHD and stroke).**

6. **Previous stroke.**

7. **Diabetes: > 20 years or with nephropathy/retinopathy.**

8. **Hypertension: > 160 mmHg systolic and/or 95 mmHg diastolic.**

9. **Focal migraine with aura (causes cerebral ischaemia, increasing the risk of stroke).**

10. **Previous deep vein thrombosis/pulmonary embolism (DVT/PE) or multiple risk factors for DVT, e.g. thrombophilia, prolonged immobilisation.**

11. **Liver disease: cirrhosis (severe decompensated disease), liver tumour, active viral hepatitis.**

12. **Breast cancer (as potentially oestrogen sensitive).**

Obstetrics

❶ The contraindications to the COC relate mainly to oestrogen, which induces a pro-thrombotic state increasing the risk of IHD, stroke and DVT/PE. There are absolute and relative contraindications to the COC and risks and benefits should be individualised for each woman. If the COC is contraindicated in a woman, she may be prescribed the progestogen-only pill (POP); however, this is still contraindicated with liver disease, undiagnosed genital tract bleeding, IHD and previous ectopic pregnancy.

Nothing in her history contraindicates the pill. She is prescribed a 3-month supply of a COC and advised on its side effects.

Q Name six *minor* side effects that Ageeth may experience   **3 marks**

1. **Depression.**

2. **Headaches.**

3. **Loss of libido.**

4. **Nausea and vomiting.**

5. **Breast tenderness.**

6. **Breakthrough bleeding/spotting (in first few cycles).**

7. **Chloasma (facial pigmentation).**

8. **Oligomenorrhoea.**

❶ Weight gain has not been shown to be associated with COC use.

❶ More serious (although rare) side effects include DVT/PE, stroke, IHD, breast and cervical cancer, gallstones and cholestatic jaundice. However, it is worth mentioning the positive side effects of the COC, including reduced risk of ovarian cancer (and cysts) and endometrial cancer (and uterine fibroids), and reduced premenstrual and dysmenorrhoea symptoms.

Q List six pieces of additional advice that you would give Ageeth   **3 marks**

1. **When to start the pill, i.e. start on day 1 of period so as to exclude pregnancy.**

Obstetrics

2. Limitations of the COC, e.g. does not protect against STIs.

3. Factors that reduce its effectiveness, e.g. if on antibiotics for < 3 weeks, if have diarrhoea or vomiting within 2 h of taking the pill or if taking liver enzyme-inducing medication (e.g. rifampicin, St John's wort, certain anticonvulsants).

4. Availability of emergency contraception.

5. Symptoms requiring immediate consultation, e.g. focal neurological signs, prolonged headache, sudden severe chest pain, shortness of breath, haemoptysis, calf pain, jaundice.

6. When you need to see her again, e.g. repeat prescription, blood pressure check.

7. Preconception advice, e.g. folate supplements, to wait for one natural period after stopping pill before attempting conception (so can accurately date pregnancy using LMP).

Several months later Ageeth attends her GUM clinic complaining of an offensive vaginal discharge.

Q List four additional clinical features that would suggest PID 2 marks

1. Bilateral lower abdominal pain and tenderness.

2. Cervical excitation, i.e. tenderness when cervix is moved on vaginal examination.

3. Adnexal tenderness on vaginal examination.

4. Pelvic mass, i.e. as a result of a pelvic abscess (woman would be systemically unwell).

5. Pyrexia.

6. Deep dyspareunia.

7. Menorrhagia.

8. Intermenstrual bleeding.

9. Dysmenorrhoea.

Obstetrics

❶ PID is typically caused by ascending genital tract infection. Infection may be asymptomatic. Acute symptomatic cases present with vaginal discharge and clinical features 1–5; chronic infection may cause vague pelvic pain with additional features 6–9. Complications include tubal infertility and ectopic pregnancy.

Q **What six questions would you ask in the sexual history?**   3 marks

1. **Characteristics of the discharge, e.g. colour, smell and duration.**

2. **Number, gender, origin and dates of sexual partners.**

3. **Whether sex was oral, vaginal and/or anal.**

4. **What contraception was used?**

5. **Previous history of STIs.**

6. **Partner's or partners' STI history including any current symptoms.**

7. **Contact details of sexual partners for contact tracing.**

8. **Human immunodeficiency virus (HIV) status (if known).**

9. **Hepatitis B virus immunisation status.**

10. **History of blood transfusion.**

❶ Baseline investigations for abnormal vaginal discharge involve: (1) speculum examination of the vagina and cervix; (2) high vaginal swab (HVS) taken from lateral vaginal walls and posterior fornix; (3) endocervical swab (for gonorrhoea and chlamydial infection); and (4) vaginal pH.

Q **List three causes of vaginal discharge**   3 marks

1. **Physiological: varying degrees of mucus discharge (leukorrhoea) during menstrual cycle, peaking around ovulation.**

2. *Trichomonas vaginalis*: **protozoan parasite that infects the vagina causing characteristic frothy, offensive, yellow discharge. Diagnosed by HVS identifying motile protozoa under microscopy. Treatment is metronidazole.**

3. *Neisseria gonorrhoeae*: **detected with endocervical swab.**

4. *Chlamydia trachomatis.*

5. *Candida albicans* (thrush): a fungus that is part of the normal vaginal flora, which may multiply (e.g. as a result of the COC, diabetes), causing a thick white discharge and severe vaginal irritation. It is diagnosed from HVS microscopy (Gram positive) and culture. Treatment is with antifungal agents, usually clotrimazole per vaginum.

6. Bacterial vaginosis (caused by abnormal vaginal bacterial flora): the most common cause of vaginal discharge, resulting in a thin greyish discharge with a fishy odour. It is diagnosed by HVS microscopy (i.e. clue cells: epithelial cells with adherent bacteria) and a raised vaginal pH (> 4.5). Treatment is metronidazole.

7. Cervical lesions (e.g. polyps): visualised on speculum examination.

8. Genital tract malignancy.

9. Foreign bodies: retained tampon or condom.

❶ Chlamydial infection is the most common STI in the UK, infecting the endocervix and causing vaginal discharge, dysuria, dyspareunia and postcoital/intermenstrual bleeding. *Chlamydia* species is an intracellular bacterium so it does not Gram stain; it is diagnosed by endocervical swab antigen testing. It can also be diagnosed by a urethral swab or a urine sample (using polymerase chain reaction [PCR] technique). Over recent years there has been a considerable rise in the incidence of chlamydial infection in the UK, leading to a major public health problem. The most prevalent age group is those aged 16–25. Early detection is crucial because it can prevent further complications of ectopic pregnancy and infertility. Treatment includes doxycycline although in pregnancy erythromycin should be used instead.

Endocervical and high vaginal swabs are taken. Microscopy reveals pink Gram-stained diplococci.

Q What is the likely cause of her vaginal discharge?   1 mark

1. *Neisseria gonorrhoeae.*

❶ *Neisseria gonorrhoeae* is a Gram-negative diplococcus (and hence it stains pink). It primarily infects the endocervical canal in women, causing an offensive vaginal discharge (although it is often asymptomatic, rarely so in men). It may infect the pharynx (causing pharyngitis) and rectum (causing proctitis) and swabs are also taken from these sites if infection is suspected. Complications include PID and (rarely) disseminated infection causing arthritis and macular rash. Amoxicillin was the treatment of choice but as a result of resistant strains cephalosporins and quinolones are more widely used. Sexual contacts should also be traced and treated.

Q List four additional tests that you would offer Ageeth   **2 marks**

1. **HIV serology: only positive 3 months after primary infection.**

2. **Syphilis serology.**

3. **Hepatitis B virus serology.**

4. **Cervical smear for cytology if not performed in previous 3 years.**

5. **Treatment follow-up to confirm eradication of infection.**

Total   **25 marks**

Obstetrics

PAEDIATRIC CASES: ANSWERS

PAEDIATRIC CASE 1

Chelsea, aged 3 months, is brought into A&E by her parents with a 2-day history of feeding difficulties preceded by coryzal symptoms. On examination she is pyrexial and appears dehydrated. Furthermore she has signs of respiratory distress with a widespread expiratory wheeze; her Sao$_2$ (on air) is 90 per cent.

Q Give six causes of wheezing in an infant   **3 marks**

1. **Virally induced wheeze.**

2. **Asthma.**

3. **Bronchiolitis.**

4. **Inhalation of a foreign body.**

5. **Croup (laryngotracheobronchitis).**

6. **Upper airway obstruction.**

7. **Gastro-oesophageal reflux.**

8. **Cardiac failure.**

9. **Cystic fibrosis.**

10. **Vascular ring.**

11. **Vocal fold dysfunction.**

12. **Tracheal or bronchial stenosis.**

❶ Wheeze is a musical sound caused by turbulent airflow through an obstructed airway. The pattern of the wheeze can be described according to:

QUESTIONS PAGES 77–80

- frequency: high or low pitched

- duration: long or short

- timing: inspiratory or expiratory

- single or multiple notes: monophonic or polyphonic.

❶ An example of a polyphonic wheeze is asthma or acute bronchospasm; a monophonic wheeze implies bronchial obstruction or structural abnormalities.

Q **List six signs of respiratory distress in an infant**   3 marks

1. **Tachypnoea (respiratory rate > 50/min).**

2. **Nasal flaring (enlargement of the opening of the nostril during breathing).**

3. **Subcostal recession.**

4. **Intercostal recession.**

5. **Supracostal recession (tracheal tug).**

6. **Chest hyperinflation.**

7. **Liver displaced inferiorly.**

8. **Cyanosis or pallor.**

9. **Use of accessory muscles, e.g. causing head bobbing.**

10. **Expiratory grunting: caused by closure of epiglottis in order to try to create positive airway pressure during expiration.**

11. **Tachycardia.**

12. **Feeding difficulties.**

Q **What is the normal heart rate and respiratory rate in infants?**   2 marks

Age	Respiratory rate (/min)	Heart rate (/min)
Infant (< 1 year)	**30–40**	**110–160**
Young child (2–5 years)	20–30	95–140
Older child (5–12 years)	20–25	80–120

ℹ Normal systolic blood pressure in infants is 70–90 mmHg.

Q List eight signs indicating dehydration in an infant 2 marks

1. **Dry tongue (< 5 per cent).**

2. **Dull, dry eyes (< 5 per cent).**

3. **Sunken anterior fontanelle (5–10 per cent).**

4. **Reduced skin turgor (5–10 per cent).**

5. **Delayed (i.e. > 2 s) capillary refill time (5–10 per cent).**

6. **Irritability (5–10 per cent).**

7. **Dry nappy, i.e. oliguria/anuria (>10 per cent).**

8. **Weak pulse (>10 per cent).**

9. **Reduced blood pressure: normal systolic BP in infant is 70–90 mmHg (> 10 per cent).**

ℹ Signs 1–2 indicate mild dehydration, i.e. < 5 per cent loss of body weight. Signs 3–6 (plus earlier signs) indicate moderate dehydration, i.e. 5–10 per cent loss of body weight. Signs 7–9 (plus earlier signs) indicate severe dehydration, i.e. > 10 per cent loss of body weight. This percentage classification is used to calculate fluid replacement requirements.

ℹ Severe dehydration can cause hypovolaemic shock and acute renal failure. Dehydration may be associated with hyper- or hyponatraemia. Hyponatraemia is associated with confusion, hypotonia and seizures. Rehydration is according to the type and severity of dehydration and can be with oral rehydration solutions, physiological saline (0.9 per cent) or half-physiological saline (0.45 per cent).

Q How are the maintenance fluid requirements of a child calculated? 2 marks

1. **They are calculated per kilogram body weight:**

   the first 10 kg: 1 L fluid/day

   the second 10 kg: add 500 mL/day (total now 1500 mL)

   above that add 20 mL/additional kg per day.

Paediatrics

253

❶ The maintenance fluid requirements per day of a 25 kg child are: 1 L (for the first 10 kg) + 500 mL (for the second 10 kg) + 100 mL (5 × 20 mL) = 1600 mL/day, i.e. 1600/24 = 66 mL/h.

❶ Fluid deficit can be calculated using the following formula:

Percentage dehydration × Weight (kg) × 10

i.e. for a 25 kg child who is 10 per cent dehydrated: 10 × 25 × 10 = 2500. This should be added to the maintenance fluid requirements to make total fluid requirements/day.

Chelsea is diagnosed with bronchiolitis and is admitted on the ward and barrier nursed to prevent spread.

Q **What are the four cardinal signs of bronchiolitis?**   **2 marks**

1. **Fever.**

2. **Wheeze.**

3. **Dry cough.**

4. **Runny nose.**

❶ Associated symptoms are: poor feeding, increased respiratory effort and apnoea in very young children (apnoea may be presenting feature in premature babies or very-low-birthweight babies). On examination there may be (although not always!) a high-pitched wheeze with inspiratory crackles. Bronchiolitis is typically preceded by a coryzal illness for 2–3 days. It mainly affects children < 2 years of age (peak incidence is 3–6 months) and is more common in the winter.

Q **List four types of patient at risk of bronchiolitis**   **2 marks**

1. **Prematurity.**

2. **Chronic lung disease: defined as O_2 therapy beyond 36 weeks' gestation.**

3. **Congenital heart disease.**

4. **Down's syndrome.**

5. **Cystic fibrosis.**

6. **Immune deficiency, e.g. severe combined immune deficiency (SCID).**

7. **Parental smoking.**

Q **What is the common cause of bronchiolitis and how is it detected?** 2 marks

1. **Respiratory syncytial virus RSV: causative agent in approximately 70 per cent of cases.**

2. **Nasopharyngeal aspirate for RSV confirmation by detection of immunofluorescent-labelled antibody.**

❶ RSV is a very common, highly contagious virus that spreads from respiratory secretions by coughing/sneezing. By 1 year of age 80 per cent of children will have been infected with RSV, of whom 20 per cent develop symptomatic disease.

❶ Other causes of bronchiolitis include adenovirus, influenza virus and parainfluenza virus.

Q **How would you manage Chelsea?** 3 marks

1. **Humidified O_2 by facemask or nasal cannulae with the aim of maintaining $Sao_2 > 92$ per cent.**

2. **Nasogastric feeding: if the infant is unable to tolerate a nasogastric tube (NGT) consider intravenous fluids (dextrose saline).**

3. **Antipyretic, e.g. paracetamol (Calpol): lowering temperature reduces the risk of dehydration and febrile convulsions.**

4. **Consider nasal suction to clear secretions if infant is showing respiratory distress.**

5. **Continuous Sao_2 monitoring: bronchiolitic infants are at risk of apnoea. Infants with $Sao_2 < 92$ per cent on air are admitted to hospital.**

❶ There is no evidence to support the use of inhaled/nebulised bronchodilators and steroids. Antibiotics are not indicated unless secondary bacterial pneumonia is suspected.

Q **What is the prophylactic antibody for RSV?** 2 marks

1. **Palivizumab.**

Paediatrics

255

❶ This is a humanised monoclonal RSV antibody. It is not recommended for routine use but should be considered in children < 1 year with significant co-morbidity (i.e. immune deficiency, extreme prematurity, chronic lung disease and acyanotic congenital heart disease). It does not prevent infection but reduces the severity of complications of RSV disease.

Q How would you monitor the effectiveness of treatment?   2 marks

1. **Respiratory rate.**

2. **Heart rate.**

3. **Temperature.**

4. **Sao₂.**

5. **Toleration of oral feeds.**

❶ Discharge criteria for bronchiolitis are temperature < 38°C, feeding adequately (> 75 per cent of usual intake), Sao_2 >94 per cent in air, respiratory rate < 50/min and heart rate < 140/min. On discharge, parents and/or carers should receive information about bronchiolitis – namely the duration of symptoms, its treatment and prognosis.

Total   **25 marks**

REFERENCE

Scottish Intercollegiate Guidelines Network (SIGN). *Bronchiolitis in Children,* **2006: www.sign.ac.uk**

Paediatrics

PAEDIATRIC CASE 2

James, aged 3 years is referred to the paediatric outpatient clinic because of poor weight gain over the last 6 months. He was born at full term weighing 3.2 kg. However, over the last 6 months his mum says that he has become irritable, his abdomen seems distended and he has lots of liquid stools that are foul smelling and difficult to flush. On examination James is pale and his abdomen protrudes. There is wasting of his muscles (especially buttocks) and his ankles seem swollen.

Q Define failure to thrive   **2 marks**

1. **Failure to thrive (FTT) is defined as poor weight gain in infants (< 1 year old) and toddlers (1–3 years) with a fall across two or more weight centile lines.**

❶ A less strict definition is 'rate of growth that does not meet the expected potential for a child of that age'. Nowadays a more parent-friendly term than failure to thrive is 'faltering growth pattern'.

❶ In order to diagnose FFT the child's weight, height and head circumference should be accurately plotted on a growth chart to assess the trend.

Q List four non-organic causes of failure to thrive   **4 marks**

1. **Inadequate food intake, e.g. as a result of insufficient food offered.**

2. **Inappropriate foods offered, e.g. too much milk or juice.**

3. **Low socioeconomic status, e.g. unable to afford a good diet.**

4. **Mechanical feeding problems, e.g. poor breast-feeding technique, oromotor dysfunction, congenital abnormalities (e.g. cleft lip, Pierre Robin syndrome)**

QUESTIONS
PAGES
81–83

5. **Emotional deprivation: disturbed parent–child relationship resulting in infant not demanding food (often accompanied by delays in development dependent on stimulation, e.g. speech).**

6. **Abuse, e.g. child neglect; rarely Munchausen syndrome by proxy, i.e. mother is deliberately underfeeding child to generate illness.**

❶ Causes of FTT can be classified as organic (underlying pathology) or non-organic (psychosocial and environmental causes). Non-organic causes account for > 95 per cent cases of FTT. Organic causes include gastro-oesophageal reflux disease (leading to poor retention of food), coeliac disease, cystic fibrosis and Crohn's disease (all causing malabsorption), and kidney and heart disease (illness-induced anorexia).

Q What is the mechanism of James's diarrhoea?   **1 mark**

1. **Malabsorption**

❶ Liquid, pale, foul smelling and difficult to flush stools (called steatorrhoea) are typically caused by malabsorption. Malabsorption is caused by a defect in the digestive process. This can be one of the following:

- Failure to produce enzymes needed to digest certain foods (lack of pancreatic enzymes in cystic fibrosis, lack of lactase in lactose intolerance)

- Failure to produce bile salt to emulsify fats as in cirrhosis and gallstone disease

- As a result of inflammation or injury to part of the intestine (such as in coeliac disease), radiation-induced injury (radiation enteritis) or inflammatory bowel disease

- Caused by abnormal gut flora as a result of bacterial overgrowth or parasite infestation.

❶ Other symptoms of malabsorption include abdominal pain, bloating and distension, which are caused by bacterial fermentation of undigested food substances producing gaseous products.

Q What is the underlying cause of James's ankle oedema?   **2 marks**

1. **Hypoproteinaemia (hypoalbuminaemia).**

Paediatrics

ⓘ Malabsorption causes failure to absorb nutrients from the diet, namely fats, carbohydrates, protein, vitamins and/or minerals. Failure to absorb protein causes oedema as a result of the reduction in plasma oncotic pressure causing a shift of fluid from the intravascular to the interstitial space. Reduced protein is also the cause of muscle wasting and atrophy found in malabsorption syndromes.

ⓘ Other manifestation of malabsorption are:

- Anaemia: caused by iron, folate and/or vitamin B_{12} deficiency

- Osteoporosis or rickets: as a result of calcium and vitamin D deficiency

- Weight loss and fatigue caused by carbohydrates, protein and fat malabsorption

- Bleeding disorders resulting from vitamin K deficiency.

As part of his investigations James is screened for coeliac disease.

Q **What is the most sensitive and specific screening test for coeliac disease?** 1 mark

1. **Endomysial antibodies (EMAs).**

ⓘ Three antibodies (i.e. endomysial, tissue transglutaminase [tTG] and anti-gliadin antibodies) can be used to screen for coeliac disease, although EMAs are the most sensitive (> 85 per cent) and specific (96–100 per cent). Endomysium is smooth muscle connective tissue. The antigen in endomysium targeted by EMA is tissue transglutaminase, which helps digest gliadin, the main peptide of gluten.

ⓘ These antibodies can also be used to assess adherence to a gluten-free diet because levels should become undetectable with dietary exclusion.

James's screening test is positive and he is referred for a jejunal biopsy, which subsequently confirms coeliac disease.

Q **List two histological changes on biopsy seen in coeliac disease** 2 marks

1. **Flat jejunal mucosa (reducing the area available for intestinal absorption).**

Paediatrics

2. **Villous atrophy.**

3. **Crypt hyperplasia caused by inflammatory cell infiltrate in the lamina propria.**

❶ Coeliac disease is an immune disorder triggered by an environmental agent (gluten). Gluten causes a T-cell-mediated inflammatory response in the proximal small bowel that damages the mucosa and leads to malabsorption. It is more common in people with autoimmune diseases (type 1 diabetes), those who have family members with coeliac disease, those with genetic conditions (Down's, Williams and Turner syndromes) and those with the HLA-DQ2/-DQ8 gene.

❶ Prevalence of coeliac disease is approximately 1 in a 100. Symptoms in children may occur around weaning (after the introduction of gluten into the diet) and the child typically presents between 1 and 3 years of age (although be aware that it can present at any age!).

Q **Which rash is associated with coeliac disease?**   2 marks

1. **Dermatitis herpetiformis.**

❶ This presents as erythematous raised patches typically on the elbows, knees and buttocks. These lesions may blister and cause pruritus. Treatment is by gluten-free diet and dapsone, but it may take months for the rash to clear.

❶ Coeliac disease can present with a wide range of symptoms and signs including diarrhoea, FTT, abdominal pain/distension, muscle wasting, irritability, anorexia, vomiting, lassitude/malaise, osteoporosis and anaemia.

Q **List three food groups that James will now have to avoid**   3 marks

1. **Wheat.**

2. **Rye.**

3. **Barley.**

4. **Oats: this is more controversial but, as most commercially available oats are contaminated with gluten, they should also be avoided.**

❶ Children should be started on a gluten-free diet only if they have their diagnosis confirmed by biopsy and never on the basis of a positive antibody test alone. Current practice is that a gluten-free diet should be adhered to for life. Gluten-free foods can be obtained on prescription and membership of the Coeliac Society should be encouraged (www.coeliac.co.uk).

❶ In addition to dietary restrictions nutritional deficiencies should be identified (including iron, folate, vitamin D and calcium) and corrected. Finally pneumococcal vaccine is now recommended in all children with coeliac disease because most patients will have some degree of hyposplenism.

Q Give three complications of coeliac disease   **3 marks**

1. **Anaemia: folate, vitamin B$_{12}$ or iron deficiency.**

2. **Small bowel non-Hodgkin's lymphoma.**

3. **Intestinal malignancies: oesophageal and large bowel squamous carcinoma, small bowel adenocarcinoma.**

4. **Osteoporosis.**

5. **Infertility.**

6. **Hyposplenism: increased risk of infections.**

❶ Benefits of a gluten-free diet include: resolution of gastrointestinal (GI) symptoms (this can be spectacular), normalisation of antibody tests and small bowel histology, reversal of bone mineralisation and infertility, and return of level of risk for intestinal malignancy to that of normal population level.

Total   **20 marks**

REFERENCE

British Society of Paediatric Gastroenterology, Hepatology and Nutrition (BSPGHAN). *Guideline for the Diagnosis and Management of Coeliac Disease in Children*, **2006. http://bspghan.org.uk/working_groups/coeliac.shtml**

Paediatrics

261

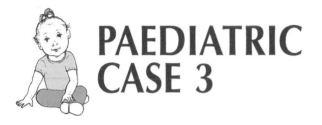

PAEDIATRIC CASE 3

Rebecca is born at 40 weeks' gestation by normal vaginal delivery weighing 3.2 kg. Her mother (gravida 1, para 1) went into labour spontaneously and labour was not prolonged. Rebecca's Apgar scores were 9 and 10 at 1 and 5 min, respectively, and she was transferred to the postnatal ward together with her mother. At the postnatal check the next day the midwife notices that Rebecca's skin and sclerae are yellow. Apart from that she appears very well and is breast-feeding satisfactorily.

Q Are you concerned about Rebecca's jaundice and briefly explain your reasoning? 2 marks

1. **Yes.**

2. **Jaundice < 24 hours after birth is always pathological.**

❶ Jaundice within 24 hours is pathological and may be the result of haemolysis or congenital infection. Bilirubin levels can rise rapidly and if unconjugated (as in haemolysis) may need aggressive treatment. Jaundice after 24 hours may be either pathological or physiological (see below).

Q Give three reasons why jaundice is common in neonates 3 marks

1. **Increased bilirubin production: compared with adults neonates have a two- to threefold increase in bilirubin production. This is because the haemoglobin concentration decreases rapidly in the first few days after birth from physiological haemolysis.**

2. **Half-life of red blood cells in neonates (70 days) is shorter than in adults (120 days).**

3. **Immaturity of hepatic bilirubin metabolism: resulting in less efficient bilirubin uptake, conjugation and excretion.**

QUESTIONS PAGES 84–86

4. **Breast-feeding: cause of jaundice in breast-fed infants is unknown although it may be related to reduced fluid intake.**

Rebecca's jaundice is investigated. Her blood results are shown in the table.

Hb (g/dL)	12.2 (range 14.5–21.5)	Rebecca's blood group	A, Rh −ve
Platelets (× 10⁹/L)	220 (range 150–400)	Maternal blood group	O, Rh −ve
MCV (fL)	112 (range 100–135)	Total serum bilirubin (μmol/L)	140 (range 3–17) (unconjugated)
WCC (× 10⁹/L)	14 (range 10–26)	CRP (mg/L)	< 10
Film	Normal RBCs	DCT	+ (mildly +ve)

Q **Give three causes of elevated *conjugated* bilirubin in neonates**   3 marks

1. **Bile duct obstruction, e.g. biliary atresia.**

2. **Congenital infections, e.g. TORCH (toxoplasmosis, other (e.g. syphilis, HIV), rubella, CMV [cytomegalovirus], herpes).**

3. **Sepsis**

4. **Neonatal hepatitis.**

5. **Inborn error of metabolism (galactosaemia, tyrosinosis).**

❶ Bilirubin is lipid soluble and must be converted into a water-soluble conjugate to be eliminated from the body. Once conjugated (with glucuronic acid in the liver) bilirubin is excreted through the bile into the small intestine and eliminated into the stool. Conjugated hyperbilirubinaemia is mostly the result of illnesses that reduce the rate of secretion of bilirubin into bile or slow down the flow of bile into the intestines (cholestasis).

❶ Unconjugated hyperbilirubinaemia occurs when there is:

- Too much bilirubin production, as in haemolysis (rhesus and ABO incompatibility, spherocytosis, G6PD [glucose-6-phosphate dehydrogenase] deficiency)

- Failure of bilirubin uptake (e.g. Gilbert's syndrome)

Paediatrics

263

- Impaired conjugation of bilirubin (e.g. Crigler–Najjar syndrome)

- Other causes such as physiological or breast milk jaundice.

Q What does the DCT detect and what does it indicate?　　2 marks

1. **The DCT (also called the direct anti-globulin test) detects the presence of antibody-coated red blood cells.**

2. **This indicates immune-mediated haemolysis, e.g. rhesus or ABO incompatibility.**

❶ A positive DCT confirms an immune aetiology, although it may be negative in ABO incompatibility.

Q From the blood results, what is the cause of Rebecca's jaundice?　　2 marks

1. **ABO incompatibility.**

❶ A moderately reduced Hb, elevated unconjugated bilirubin and a mildly positive Coombs' test are typically seen in ABO incompatibility. This is confirmed by maternal blood group O and neonatal blood group A. The mother will have circulating anti-A (and anti-B) IgG antibodies, which can cross the placenta and cause immune-mediated haemolysis.

❶ Rhesus incompatibility is not possible as both Rebecca and her mum are rhesus negative. The blood film is normal making spherocytosis unlikely (although lack of spherocytes does not altogether exclude spherocytosis).

❶ Jaundice is visible when bilirubin levels reach > 40 μmol/L.

Q What is your initial management?　　1 mark

1. **Take serial measurements of bilirubin (every 2–4 hours depending on how steeply levels are rising) and plot on a chart.**

❶ Bilirubin levels tend to increase linearly, so plotting serial concentrations on a chart can be used to predict when phototherapy or exchange transfusion may be required. The decision to start phototherapy depends on level of serum bilirubin, gestational age of the baby and rate of rise of bilirubin.

Q How does phototherapy work?   1 mark

1. **Light (blue and white light) converts unconjugated bilirubin by photodegradation into harmless water-soluble metabolites, which are excreted in bile and urine.**

   If unconjugated bilirubin reaches high levels (> 360 μmol/L) it can become neurotoxic.

Q What is this neurotoxicity called?   1 mark

1. **Kernicterus.**

❶ Unconjugated bilirubin is lipid soluble and, when levels exceed the binding capacity of albumin, bilirubin can cross the blood–brain barrier. Deposition of bilirubin in the basal ganglia and brain stem has severe neurological consequences that may even be permanent.

Q Give three clinical features of this   3 marks

1. **Sleepiness.**

2. **Poor feeding.**

3. **Hypotonia.**

4. **Poor Moro response.**

5. **High-pitched cry.**

6. **Irritability.**

7. **Seizures.**

8. **Arched back (opisthotonus).**

❶ Early signs of kernicterus typically happen 3–4 days after birth.

Q Give two long-term complications of this   2 marks

1. **Learning difficulties.**

2. **Enamel dysplasia.**

Paediatrics

265

3. **Cerebral palsy, e.g. dyskinesia cerebral palsy as a result of bilirubin deposition in the basal ganglia (typically causing ataxia and choreoathetosis).**

4. **Sensorineural deafness: all babies treated for jaundice undergo hearing tests (brain-stem-evoked audiometry) before discharge.**

❶ These complications appear around 18–24 months.

Fortunately for Rebecca, phototherapy is successful and she joins her new family at home 4 days later on oral folic acid. She is followed up 2 weeks later in outpatients for a repeat FBC to ensure that late haemolysis is not occurring.

Total   **20 marks**

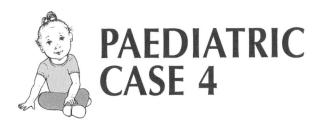

PAEDIATRIC CASE 4

Sarah is a 15-month-old, happy toddler who has just started to walk. Mum has noticed recently that when Sarah walks she seems to drag her left foot. Sarah appears unaware of this and does not complain of any pain. She was born full term with a normal vaginal delivery and there were no antenatal or postnatal problems.

Q With regard to her motor milestones, at what ages would you expect Sarah to do the following?   **7 marks**

1. **Crawl: 8–9 months.**

2. **Walk: 12–18 months.**

3. **Run: 1.5–2 years.**

4. **Kick a ball: 2–2.5 years.**

5. **Ride a tricycle: 3 years.**

6. **Hop on one foot: 4 years.**

7. **Climb stairs adult fashion: 5 years.**

🛈 Developmental milestones are divided into four areas:

1. Gross motor

2. Fine motor and vision

3. Speech, language and hearing

4. Social, emotional and behaviour.

Paediatrics

❶ There is variation in the rate at which children develop but there are limit ages by which a child should have acquired certain skills. Further assessment is indicated if the child falls outside these limit ages. Most common causes of developmental delay are cerebral palsy, primary muscle disorders and global developmental delay.

❶ A limb is considered a deviation from the normal gait pattern for that child's age and development.

Q **Name four pathological gaits in children** 2 marks

1. **Trendelenburg's (or waddling) gait: as a result of weakness of abductor muscles causing downward tilting of the hip on the opposite side, with the patient having to swing that leg round to make a step. Causes include developmental dysplasia of the hip, leg calf Perthes' disease and slipped capital femoral epiphysis (CFE).**

2. **Antalgic gait: adopted because of (hip) pain. Patient leans to side of pain in the hip and takes short, heavy, quick steps on that side and longer steps on the unaffected side. Causes include infection, trauma, slipped femoral epiphysis, limb deformity, arthritis.**

3. **Ataxic gait: wide-based gait caused by loss of proprioception or cerebellar disturbance, e.g. in ataxic cerebral palsy.**

4. **Foot-drop gait: difficulty with dorsiflexion of the foot. The knee is raised high to lift the foot off the ground, which otherwise scrapes the floor, e.g. in cerebral palsy or peroneal muscle atrophy.**

5. **Spastic gait: stiff legs with unbalanced coordination of different muscle groups, e.g. knees and thighs are crossed (termed scissoring); foot is often dragged along the floor. Caused by CNS lesions, e.g. cerebral palsy.**

Q List six questions that you want to ask Mum 3 marks

1. **How long has she been limping, e.g. acute onset in trauma and septic arthritis?**

2. **Any history of trauma (also be aware of non-accidental injury)?**

3. **Can she weight bear, e.g. not weight bearing is seen in septic arthritis?**

Paediatrics

4. **Does she appear to be in pain? If so, when is the pain worst? Pain in the morning may suggest rheumatoid conditions; night pain (especially if it wakes the child from sleep) points more towards a neoplastic process.**

5. **Any weakness in the leg, e.g. neuromuscular conditions?**

6. **Are any other joints affected? May suggest a viral illness, rheumatological conditions.**

7. **Any associated features: fever or weight loss?**

8. **Is she able to do her normal activities?**

❶ Be aware of referred pain, e.g. hip pathology causing knee pain, so always examine the whole limb.

Q **What is your differential diagnosis?**   2 marks

1. **Developmental dysplasia of the hip.**

2. **Trauma: fractures, sprain, contusion.**

3. **Infectious: osteomyelitis, septic arthritis.**

4. **Neoplastic: osteogenic sarcoma.**

5. **Neuromuscular: cerebral palsy (in boys also consider Duchenne's muscular dystrophy).**

6. **Rheumatological disorders.**

Q **Which diagnosis needs immediate intervention?**   1 mark

1. **Septic arthritis.**

❶ Septic arthritis typically infects the hip joint in young children and knees in older children and adults. In most cases of septic arthritis in children, the child is younger than 3 years. Clinical manifestations include fever, joint effusion, raised inflammatory markers, and refusal to move the affected limb or weight bear.

Paediatrics

269

❶ If an effusion is present, which can be confirmed with ultrasonography, the key investigation is joint aspiration for microscopy, culture and sensitivities. Common causative organisms include *Staphylococcus aureus*, *Haemophilus influenzae* and group B streptococcus. Intravenous antibiotics should be started immediately after joint aspiration because joint destruction can be very rapid and lead to permanent loss of function.

Q **What two manoeuvres can you do to test for congenital hip problems in neonates?** 1 mark

1. **Barlow test: attempt to dislocate an unstable hip. The thigh is taken between examiner's thumb and fingers (middle finger over greater trochanter) and is adducted and pressed posteriorly. If positive, dislocation is felt as the femoral head slips out of the acetabulum.**

2. **Ortolani test: this is the opposite of the Barlow test because it attempts to reduce a dislocated hip. The neonate's thigh is taken between thumb and fingers and abducted and pulled anteriorly. If positive the examiner will feel a 'clunk' as the femoral head is reduced into the acetabulum**

❶ One in 100 newborns has an unstable hip, i.e. developmental dysplasia of the hip (DDH), which if untreated may lead to pain, stiffness (causing problems with gait) and arthritis. Risk factors include positive family history, ligamentous laxity, primagravida, breech presentation and oligohydramnios. In addition to the above Barlow or Ortolani test, look for discrepancy in leg length and asymmetry of leg creases on examination. If DDH is suspected, ultrasonography of the hip is recommended to assess hip stability and acetabular development. Treatment depends on the child's age at diagnosis: the aim is to reduce dislocation and maintain reduction of the hip. Rarely reduction may cause avascular necrosis of the capital femoral epiphysis secondary to compression of the cartilage.

Your next patient also presents with a limp: a 12-year-old boy whose weight lies on the 90th centile and who has been complaining for several weeks of an intermittent limp and knee pain making cycling painful.

Q **What is the most likely diagnosis from this history?** 1 mark

1. **Slipped femoral epiphysis (SFE).**

❶ A limp (antalgic gait) together with thigh, knee or groin pain (although not hip pain) for several weeks in a pubescent, obese male is most likely to be caused by SFE. It is defined as inferior and posterior slippage of the proximal femoral epiphysis through the growth plate. It can be classified into stable (chronic symptoms) and unstable (acute presentation) depending on the degree of disruption between capital femoral epiphysis (CFE) and femoral neck.

Q **What is the typical finding on examination of the hip?**   **2 marks**

1. **Decreased internal rotation.**

❶ The first sign is decreased internal rotation of the hip, followed by increased external rotation and flexion and abduction of the hip (sometimes to a fixed position). With time a discrepancy in leg length may develop together with atrophy of the thigh muscles.

❶ Treatment depends on the severity of the slippage but in unstable and acute cases of SFE internal fixation is necessary. Complications of SFE include avascular necrosis and chondrolysis (destruction of the articular cartilage of the hip joint).

Q **Which other hip pathology in a child is associated with avascular necrosis?**   **1 mark**

1. **Leg calf Perthes' disease (LCPD).**

❶ LCPD is idiopathic avascular necrosis of the CFE. It is caused by interruption of the blood supply to the CFE, leading to osteonecrosis of the ossification centre of the femoral epiphysis. In some children revascularisation and subsequent normal bone growth occurs whereas in others LCPD develops. It is more common in boys (aged 2–12 years). Clinical presentation is with a limp, hip or groin pain, muscle spasm and decreased range of movement (internal rotation and abduction). Radiographs are necessary to determine the extent of damage to the CFE. Treatment is conservative with the aim of limiting the deformity of the femoral head. The main complication is development of osteoarthritis in adulthood.

Total   **20 marks**

Paediatrics

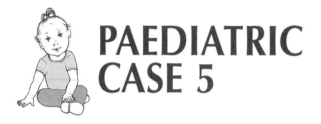

PAEDIATRIC CASE 5

Nathan is an 11-month-old infant who has been referred to the paediatric assessment unit with a history of irritability and inconsolable crying for the last 8 hours. His mother has noted that he will settle down for a few minutes but then wake up and cry loudly, drawing his legs up to his abdomen. There is no fever, vomiting or diarrhoea. His bowels were last open yesterday and his stools were normal. Past medical history is unremarkable except that Nathan is recovering from gastroenteritis and remains off his feed.

Q List five causes of inconsolable crying in an infant   **5 marks**

1. Constipation.

2. Cows' milk protein intolerance/lactose intolerance.

3. Gastro-oesophageal reflux.

4. Infantile colic.

5. Volvulus.

6. Intussusception.

7. Foreign body in the eye/corneal abrasion.

8. Hair tourniquet (a loose hair tightly wrapped around a body part cutting off the circulation, e.g. toe or finger).

9. Urinary tract infection.

10. Otitis media.

11. Rectal fissure.

12. Testicular torsion.

13. Meningitis.

QUESTIONS
PAGES
90–92

Paediatrics

14. Trauma, e.g. fracture, including non-accidental injury.

15. Nappy rash.

Q Define infantile colic

2 marks

1. **Infantile colic is unexplained crying in an otherwise healthy and well-fed infant under the age of 3 months.**

❶ It is defined as crying for more than 3 hours per day, occurring more than 3 days per week and persisting for longer than 3 weeks (Wessel's criteria).

❶ Infantile colic is common (up to 25 per cent of infants may suffer from it at some point) and typically starts at 2 weeks of age and is often resolved by 4 months. Attacks typically happen late afternoon/evening. They are characterised by the infant pulling his legs against his abdomen with paroxysmal episodes of screaming. Associated features may be a flushed face, clenched fists and a furrowed brow. Infantile colic is a diagnosis of exclusion and the aetiology of it remains unclear. Treatment is not usually necessary or effective.

Nathan is alert, pink and well perfused. His abdomen is not distended, and is soft with normal bowel sounds and a palpable mass in the right upper quadrant.

Q What is intussusception?

1 mark

1. **Intussusception is the telescoping (folding into itself) of one proximal segment of the bowel into another more distal segment.**

❶ Intussusception is the leading cause of intestinal obstruction in children aged 3 months to 6 years (most commonly aged 3–12 months). It is more common in males and is a life-threatening condition. The mortality rate is about 2 per cent (if treated) but if left untreated it is fatal in almost all cases.

Q In which part of the bowel does intussusception most commonly occur?

1 mark

1. **Terminal ileum: the terminal part of the ileum moves into the colon through the ileocaecal valve. This is called ileocolic intussusception.**

Paediatrics

273

❶ Other types of intussusception include: ileo-ileal (small intestines loop into themselves) and colocolic (large bowel moves into itself).

Q Name four predisposing factors for intussusception   **4 marks**

❶ Intussusception is thought to be the result of abnormalities in the intestinal wall that may cause some obstruction of the bowel which may initiate the process of intussusception.

1. **Cystic fibrosis: thought to be related to faecal overloading in which a faecal bolus may adhere to the intestinal wall and thereby obstruct the bowel.**

2. **Henoch–Schönlein purpura (HSP): may cause small bowel haematomas (bruises) in the intestinal wall.**

3. **Viral illnesses, e.g. gastroenteritis: lymph nodes in the intestinal wall (called Peyer's patches) become swollen and cause a thickening of the intestinal wall.**

4. **Foreign body.**

5. **Other conditions causing abnormalities of the bowel wall, e.g. Meckel's diverticulum, intestinal polyp (e.g. Peutz–Jeghers syndrome, familial polyposis coli).**

6. **Post-abdominal surgery: trauma to the intestinal wall.**

Q Name six features of intussusception   **3 marks**

1. **Paroxysmal severe intermittent abdominal pain (child draws up legs).**

2. **Stool mixed with blood and mucus (referred to as 'red currant jelly' stool): a late sign.**

3. **A sausage-shaped mass in the abdomen (typically right upper quadrant).**

4. **Distended abdomen.**

5. **Vomiting that may become bilious.**

6. **Diarrhoea (loose watery stools).**

7. **Shock: as a result of third space fluid loss in the gut.**

Intussusception causes compression of blood vessels in the involved part of the bowel, which reduces the blood supply, leading to venous obstruction and ischaemia. This causes oedema of the bowel wall, bleeding ('red current jelly' stools) and disrupted peristalsis. If untreated, this will finally result in necrosis and perforation of the bowel wall.

Suspecting that Nathan has intussusception, you request an abdominal ultrasound scan, shown below.

Q

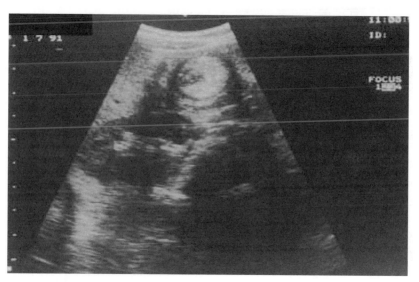

Q What does the ultrasound show?   **2 marks**

1. Doughnut or target sign appearance.

 Ultrasound scan may show a classic doughnut or target sign appearance, i.e. alternating hypoechoic and echogenic bowel wall representing the 'loop within a loop' characteristic of intussusception.

 Abdominal radiograph may show distended small bowel and absence of gas in the distal colon. Radiographs are usually, however, reserved for when perforation is suspected.

Paediatrics

Q How would you treat intussusception in Nathan? 2 marks

1. **Radiological reduction via an air or barium enema. The air increases the pressure within the bowel, which may unfold the affected part of the intestine.**

ⓘ This is successful in over 75 per cent of patients (if done early enough), although it should be performed only in the absence of peritonitis. After successful reduction, admission to the ward is usually necessary as a result of the high recurrence rate. Surgical reduction (manual unfolding out of the looped parts of bowel) is indicated when peritonitis is suspected, or when the enema has failed and/or the intussusception is present for more than 24 hours.

Total **20 marks**

RENAL CASES:
ANSWERS

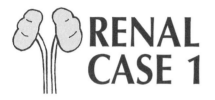# RENAL
CASE 1

Shelia, a 49-year-old woman, is investigated for malaise and fatigue by her GP. Her current medications are insulin (for type 1 diabetes), ACE inhibitor (for hypertension) and NSAID (for chronic back pain). Her blood results are shown in the table.

Hb (g/dL)	9.2	Na$^+$ (mmol/L)	136
MCV (fL)	86	K$^+$ (mmol/L)	5.7
WCC (× 10^9/L)	5.2	Urea (mmol/L)	27
Platelets (× 10^9/L)	280	Creatinine (μmol/L)	245
Glucose (mmol/L)	18.7	Adjusted Ca^{2+} (mmol/L)	1.82
HbA1c (%)	9.2	PO$_4^{3-}$ (mmol/L)	2.72

Q How much fluid is filtered through the glomerulus each day?   1 mark

1. Approximately 180 L/day, i.e. 125 mL/min × 60 (min) × 24 (h).

❶ Chronic renal failure, defined as progressive and usually irreversible impairment in renal function, is classified according to the reduction in glomerular filtration rate (GFR); the associated serum creatinine levels are as shown in the table.

Grade	GFR (mL/min)	Serum creatinine (μmol/L)
Normal	≈125	70–150
Mild	20–50	150–300
Moderate	10–20	300–700
Severe	< 10	> 700

Renal

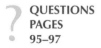**QUESTIONS**
PAGES
95–97

❶ The GFR can be calculated by measuring either clearance of intravenous inulin (which is freely filtered at the glomerulus but neither secreted nor reabsorbed by the tubules) or 24-hour urinary creatinine clearance.

❶ Refer to Appendix 3 in the *British National Formulary* (BNF) for advice on adjusting drug doses according to grade of CRF.

Q **Outline four functions of the kidney**   **4 marks**

1. **Excretion of waste products including drugs by glomerular filtration and active tubular secretion.**

2. **Fluid and electrolyte balance.**

3. **Acid:base balance: secrete H⁺ ions and reabsorb/synthesise HCO$_3^-$.**

4. **Gluconeogenesis: during fasting state.**

5. **Endocrine function.**

6. **Production of erythropoietin (see below).**

7. **Conversion of 25-hydroxy-vitamin D (25-OH-D) to 1,25-dihydroxy-vitamin D [1,25-(OH)$_2$-D] (calcitriol), the active form of vitamin D (see below).**

8. **Control of blood pressure: secretion of renin, which activates the renin–angiotensin pathway.**

Q **List three blood tests suggestive of CRF**   **3 marks**

❶ Shelia has renal failure as indicated by her raised urea (normal range 2.5–6.7 mmol/L) and creatinine (normal range 70–120 µmol/L). The following blood tests suggest chronic, as opposed to acute, renal failure:

1. **Normochromic/normocytic anaemia: Hb < 11.0 g/dL.**

2. **Hypocalcaemia: reduced adjusted calcium (2.12–2.65 mmol/L).**

3. **Hyperphosphataemia: raised phosphate (0.8–1.45 mmol/L).**

❶ Previous abnormal U&Es and small kidneys on ultrasonography also suggest CRF. However, it should be recognised that hypocalcaemia and hyperphosphataemia may also occur in ARF and anaemia may be associated with conditions causing ARF.

Q What is the likely cause of Sheila's anaemia?　　　　　1 mark

1. Erythropoietin (EPO) deficiency.

🛈 The kidneys release EPO to stimulate erythropoiesis in the bone marrow. CRF causes a deficiency in EPO resulting in anaemia. This is corrected by excluding other causes (e.g. iron and folate deficiency) and giving EPO. Blood transfusions should be avoided because it increases the risk of HLA sensitisation and hence tissue rejection in renal transplantation.

Q Name two factors that might be contributing to her renal failure　　2 marks

1. Poorly controlled diabetes (as indicated by HbA1c > 7 per cent): causing diabetic nephropathy.

2. Hypertension: causing hypertensive nephropathy.

3. ACE inhibitors: may cause *acute* renal failure as a result of reduced glomerular filtration pressure in patients with renal arterial disease.

4. NSAIDs: analgesic nephropathy.

🛈 Complications of hypertension and diabetes include CRF, the risk of which is reduced by tight control (other causes of CRF include glomerulonephritis, obstructive uropathy and polycystic kidneys). Although ACE inhibitors may cause ARF, they have been shown to reduce the rate of progression of renal failure in patients with diabetes (and should be started in all patients with diabetes who have microalbuminuria, even if normotensive).

Q List four *systemic* causes of pruritus　　　　　2 marks

🛈 The causes of pruritus can be classified as local (e.g. eczema, infestation) and systemic:

1. CRF (uraemia).

2. Jaundice (caused by bile salts).

3. Polycythaemia ruba vera: especially after a hot bath.

4. Iron-deficient anaemia.

5. Hypothyroidism.

6. **Cancer, e.g. lymphoma (B symptoms).**

7. **Drugs, e.g. combined oral contraceptive (COC), morphine.**

❶ CRF may cause a range of symptoms including malaise, lethargy, nocturia and polyuria (as a result of impaired concentrating ability), peripheral/pulmonary oedema caused by salt and water retention, pruritus, bone pain (see below), nausea and vomiting, restless leg syndrome, paraesthesiae caused by peripheral neuropathy and/or hypocalcaemia, and symptoms of anaemia.

Shelia is referred to a nephrologist for her CRF and is kept under review for progression of her disease and to prevent or treat any complications.

Q List two treatments to prevent renal bone disease   **2 marks**

❶ Renal bone disease (osteodystrophy) is prevented by aggressively treating hypocalcaemia and hyperphosphataemia by:

1. **Dietary phosphate restriction, e.g. less milk, cheese, eggs.**

2. **Phosphate binders: use of calcium-containing phosphate binders is often limited by causing hypercalcaemia; newer treatments, including sevelamer, cause fewer side effects.**

3. **Alfacalcidol or calcitrol to correct 'activated' vitamin D deficiency plus calcium supplements.**

❶ Renal bone disease is caused by reduced renal phosphate excretion resulting in hyperphosphataemia, which in turn stimulates parathyroid hormone (PTH) release. There is also reduced vitamin D activation resulting in reduced dietary Ca^{2+} absorption (causing hypocalcaemia) and increased PTH release. PTH acts to promote resorption of bone Ca^{2+} (it also causes reabsorption of PO_4^{3-}), as well as promoting renal Ca^{2+} reabsorption (and renal PO_4^{3-} excretion) so as to oppose any hypocalcaemia, ultimately causing bone disease.

Renal

❶ Treatment of other complications of CRF include low dietary potassium, e.g. avoid bananas (in treatment of hyperkalaemia), bicarbonate supplements (in severe metabolic acidosis), sodium/fluid restriction (in treatment of fluid overload and hypertension) and low protein diet to reduce rate of urea production (in treatment of severe uraemic symptoms).

Q How would you monitor the effectiveness of such treatment?   **1 mark**

1. Monitor PTH levels.

❶ PTH is measured regularly to assess whether hyperparathyroidism is being effectively suppressed by treating hypocalcaemia and hyperphosphataemia.

A graph of Shelia's reciprocal plasma creatinine against time is shown.

RENAL FUNCTION

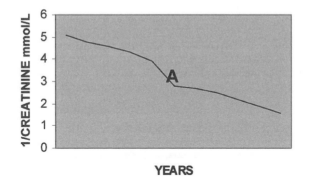

Q Give four possible causes for the sharp decline at time A   **4 marks**

❶ Renal function is monitored by reciprocal plots of plasma creatinine. Normally the decline is linear so any rapid decline needs investigating to slow down the ultimate progression to end-stage renal failure (ESRF) and dialysis. Causes of rapid decline include:

1. Uncontrolled hypertension.

2. Uncontrolled diabetes.

3. **Infection.**

4. **Dehydration.**

5. **Nephrotoxic drugs, e.g. NSAIDs.**

6. **Urinary tract obstruction.**

7. **Hypercalcaemia.**

ⓘ The decision to start dialysis depends on GFR (< 10 mL/min), complications (e.g. refractory hyperkalaemia) and/or presence of severe uraemic symptoms. The two forms of dialysis are haemodialysis and peritoneal dialysis. In haemodialysis blood is pumped through a semipermeable membrane, which allows molecules to diffuse across into the dialysis fluid down their concentration gradient. Peritoneal dialysis is simpler: dialysis fluid is introduced into the peritoneal cavity using the peritoneal membrane as the semipermeable membrane. The fluid is changed regularly to repeat the process.

Total   **20 marks**

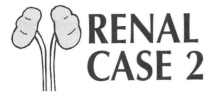# RENAL
CASE 2

Christopher, a 74-year-old man, is admitted with a 2-day history of worsening oliguria and general malaise. On examination he is hypotensive, pyrexial and clinically dehydrated. His admission U&Es are: Na⁺ 133 mmol/L, K⁺ 6.7 mmol/L, urea 41 mmol/L and creatinine 443 μmol/L. With regard to his past medical history, he is normally fit and well, taking ibuprofen for back pain and an ACE inhibitor for hypertension.

Q **List two causes each of pre-renal, renal and post-renal failure**　　　**6 marks**

Pre-renal failure:

1. **Any cause of hypovolaemia, e.g. haemorrhage.**

2. **Sepsis.**

3. **Decreased cardiac output, e.g. heart failure.**

4. **Renal artery stenosis.**

5. **Drugs, i.e. NSAIDs and ACE inhibitors, decrease renal blood flow (see below).**

❶ Pre-renal failure is the result of impaired renal perfusion as a result hypotension or hypovolaemia.

Renal failure:

1. **Acute tubular necrosis (ATN).**

2. **Nephrotoxins, e.g. NSAIDs, gentamicin.**

3. **Pyelonephritis.**

4. **Glomerulonephritis (GN): immune complex-mediated damage to the glomerulus.**

? QUESTIONS
PAGES
98–100

5. **Rhabdomyolysis (causing myoglobinuria), e.g. after crush injury, drug overdose.**

6. **Myeloma.**

7. **Urate nephropathy: tumour lysis syndrome complicating chemotherapy in haematological malignancies.**

8. **Hepatorenal syndrome: renal failure secondary to liver failure.**

9. **Malignant hypertension.**

❶ ATN is a result of pre-renal failure sufficient to cause ischaemic injury to renal tubules (ATN and pre-renal failure account for > 80 per cent of cases of ARF).

Post-renal failure:

1. **Urinary stone disease.**

2. **Benign prostatic hypertrophy (BPH).**

3. **Prostatic carcinoma.**

4. **Pelvic (e.g. bladder) or abdominal tumours.**

5. **Retroperitoneal fibrosis, e.g. methyldopa, β blockers.**

❶ Post-renal failure (obstructive nephropathy) is caused by obstruction to the renal tract anywhere from the calyces to the external urethral orifice. Although typically subacute or chronic, it is treated as ARF because it is (partially) reversible on relief of obstruction, e.g. by catheterisation, nephrostomy.

Q **What test can be used to distinguish between pre-renal failure and ATN?**

1 mark

1. **Urinary sodium: < 20 mmol/L (pre-renal); > 40 mmol/L (ATN).**

2. **Urinary osmolality: > 500 mosmol/L (pre-renal); < 350 mosmol/L (ATN).**

❶ Low urinary sodium indicates that the tubules are able to reabsorb sodium as in pre-renal failure; high urine osmolality indicates that the tubules are able to reabsorb water under the influence of antidiuretic hormone (ADH) and again suggests pre-renal failure. Higher urinary sodium and low osmolality suggest ATN (although in the presence of diuretic therapy these results can be misleading).

❶ Other investigations in ARF include (depending on clinical indication):

- Urine dipstick (nitrites, leukocytes, haematuria, protein), microscopy (e.g. red blood cell [RBC] casts, white blood cell [WBC] casts) and culture. Nitrites/leukocytes indicate a urinary tract infection (UTI); WBC casts indicate pyelonephritis. Haematuria/proteinuria may indicate GN; RBC casts indicate glomerular bleeding, e.g. as seen in GN.

- U&Es, full blood count (FBC), liver function tests (LFTs).

- Urate

- Creatine kinase (CK): ↑↑ rhabdomyolysis.

- Serum/urinary electrophoresis: myeloma screen.

- Immunology screen (if suggestive of GN): anti-nuclear antibodies (ANA), anti-neutrophil cytoplasmic antibody (ANCA), complement (↓ in systemic lupus erythematosus [SLE]), anti-glomerular basement membrane (GBM) antibodies (Goodpasture's syndrome).

- Arterial blood gases (ABGs): e.g. metabolic acidosis.

- Blood cultures.

- Kidney ureters bladder (KUB) ultrasonography: to exclude post-renal failure.

- Chest radiograph: pneumonia (source of infection), pulmonary oedema.

- ECG: e.g. hyperkalaemic changes.

Christopher is diagnosed with ARF secondary to sepsis. He is resuscitated with intravenous crystalloid, started on broad-spectrum antibiotics and his nephrotoxic drugs are stopped.

Q Outline how ACE inhibitors and NSAIDs cause ARF   **2 marks**

1. **ACE inhibitors: cause pre-renal failure (particularly in presence of renal arterial disease) as a result of *efferent* arteriole vasodilatation, thereby reducing glomerular filtration pressure.**

2. **NSAIDs can cause both pre-renal failure and renal failure:**

   – pre-renal failure: reduced glomerular filtration pressure as a result of inhibition of prostaglandin-mediated *afferent* arteriole vasodilatation.

287

– renal failure: direct nephrotoxin.

❶ The management of ARF involves:

• Monitoring of fluid balance, i.e. fluid balance charts, insertion of urinary catheter ± insertion of central venous pressure (CVP) line

• Fluid resuscitation if hypovolaemic and hypotensive; if hypotensive despite adequate fluid resuscitation may require colloid ± inotropes

• Treating the underlying cause, e.g. antibiotics if septic, stopping nephrotoxic drugs

• Management of potential complications (see below).

Appropriate investigations are taken including an ECG, as shown.

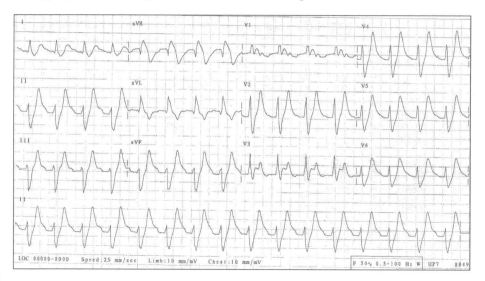

Q Give two ECG changes associated with hyperkalaemia   **1 mark**

1. **Tall, tented T waves.**

2. **Small (or absent) P waves.**

3. **Widened QRS complex.**

❶ Hyperkalaemia causes hyperpolarisation of cell membranes causing reduced cardiac excitability predisposing to arrhythmias. It requires urgent treatment if > 6.5 mmol/L or associated with the above ECG changes.

Q List four causes of hyperkalaemia   2 marks

❶ Hyperkalaemia is caused by either increased cellular release or failure of excretion. Increased cellular release may occur in:

1. **Metabolic acidosis, e.g. diabetic ketoacidosis (DKA).**

2. **Cell lysis, e.g. rhabdomyolysis, blood transfusion.**

3. **Digoxin toxicity: caused by inhibition of Na^+/K^+ pump.**

4. **Artefactual: haemolysis of blood sample.**

❶ Failure of excretion may occur in:

1. **Renal failure: both ARF and CRF.**

2. **K^+-sparing diuretics, e.g. spironolactone.**

3. **ACE inhibitors: inhibit aldosterone-mediated K^+ excretion.**

4. **Addison's disease, i.e. aldosterone deficiency.**

5. **Metabolic acidosis: H^+ competes with K^+ for excretion in the distal convoluted tubule.**

❶ K^+ and H^+ ions compete with each other for exchange of Na^+ across cellular membranes (Na^+ is pumped out) and in the distal convoluted tubule (where Na^+ is reabsorbed). Thus, in metabolic acidosis, increased H^+ will compete with K^+ for renal excretion and intracellular uptake, causing hyperkalaemia.

Q How would you treat life-threatening hyperkalaemia?   3 marks

1. **Intravenous calcium gluconate (10 mL of 10 per cent) if ECG changes: cardioprotective (stabilises the cardiac membranes), although does not reduce serum potassium concentrations.**

2. **Intravenous glucose (50 mL of 50 per cent dextrose) and insulin (10–16 U Actrapid): insulin promotes cellular uptake of K^+ by stimulating the Na^+/K^+ ATPase (glucose to counteract the effects of insulin); nebulised β_2 agonists also drive K^+ into cells.**

3. **Intravenous bicarbonate if severe metabolic acidosis (see above).**

4. **Calcium resonium (oral or rectal): only treatment that actually removes potassium from body.**

289

❶ If refractory hyperkalaemia consider renal replacement therapy (see below).

Q List four indications for renal replacement therapy   **4 marks**

1. **Severe uraemic symptoms, e.g. uraemic encephalopathy.**

2. **Uraemic complications, e.g. pericarditis.**

3. **Refractory hyperkalaemia.**

4. **Severe metabolic acidosis.**

5. **Refractory pulmonary oedema: if fluid overloaded give intravenous furosemide (250 mg over 1 h).**

6. **Removal of drugs causing ARF.**

❶ If the above complications of ARF are refractory to medical treatment the patient may require renal replacement therapy, e.g. on the intensive care unit (ICU), while awaiting recovery of renal function. Renal replacement therapy includes dialysis and haemofiltration.

Christopher's blood pressure and urine output respond to fluid resuscitation and his U&Es subsequently indicate recovery of his renal function.

Q Name two early complications following recovery from ATN   **1 mark**

❶ Although pre-renal failure is rapidly reversed by correction of the underlying cause (as in Christopher's case), recovery of ATN typically takes days to weeks. In the early stages of recovery there may be a diuretic phase where, as a result of earlier recovery of glomerular function, the GFR exceeds renal tubular reabsorption causing:

1. **Hyponatraemia.**

2. **Hypokalaemia**

3. **Hypovolaemia.**

Total   **20 marks**

290

Renal

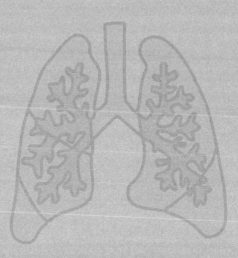

RESPIRATORY CASES: ANSWERS

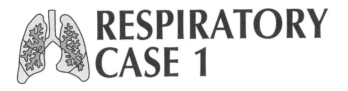 # RESPIRATORY
CASE 1

*Lucy, a 21-year-old with asthma, presents to A&E with a 2-day
history of increased shortness of breath, wheeze and cough.
On examination her pulse is 125 beats/min, blood pressure
130/80 mmHg, respiratory rate 30/min, and there is widespread
bilateral expiratory wheeze and reduced air entry throughout.*

Q What three brief questions would you ask?   3 marks

1. **Ask about usual treatments.**

2. **Best peak expiratory flow (PEF): used to assess severity/effect of treatment.**

3. **Previous admissions to hospital for acute attack including transfer to an intensive care unit (ICU); this may give an indication of the potential severity of her asthma.**

❶ The only investigations needed before *immediate treatment* are PEF (although the patient may be too ill) and pulse oximetry (Sao_2).

Q List three criteria used to indicate a severe asthma attack   3 marks

1. **Cannot complete sentences.**

2. **Respiratory rate > 25/min.**

3. **Pulse rate > 110 beats/min.**

4. **PEF < 50 per cent of predicted or best.**

Q List three criteria used to indicate a life-threatening asthma attack   3 marks

1. **Silent chest, cyanosis or poor respiratory effort.**

2. **Exhaustion, confusion or coma.**

QUESTIONS
PAGES
103–105

3. Bradycardia (heart rate [HR] < 60 beats/min) or hypotension (systolic BP < 90 mmHg).

4. PEF < 33 per cent of predicted or best.

5. Sao_2 < 92 per cent.

❶ If there are any life-threatening features warn the ICU because the patient may require transfer there for respiratory support including intubation (similarly warn the ICU if the patient has been admitted to the ICU with previous asthma attacks).

Q **What is your immediate management in *severe* asthma?**   3 marks

1. Sit patient upright and give high-flow (40–60 per cent) O_2: CO_2 retention is not usually aggravated by O_2 therapy in asthma.

2. Nebulised salbutamol (5 mg) and ipratropium bromide (500 µg).

3. Oral prednisolone (40–50 mg) or intravenous hydrocortisone (200 mg).

❶ If there are any life-threatening features give intravenous magnesium sulphate (1.2–2 g over 20 min).

❶ Intravenous aminophylline was commonly used in the past but does not usually produce additional benefit in patients who have already received β_2 agonists and steroids. Side effects include cardiac arrhythmias and, as such, treatment should be started only by a senior clinician.

Q **Other than in life-threatening asthma, when else is intravenous magnesium sulphate used?**   1 mark

1. In the treatment of eclamptic seizures: 4–6 g intravenous infusion.

2. In the treatment of ventricular arrhythmias, in particular torsade de pointes.

❶ Torsade de pointes is ventricular tachycardia (VT) with varying axis. It is caused by a prolonged Q–T interval (e.g. inherited, electrolyte disturbance such as ↓ K^+, Mg^{2+}, Ca^{2+}, and drugs such as anti-arrhythmic drugs) and may predispose to ventricular fibrillation (VF) arrest. Treatment involves stopping any causative drugs and giving 8 mmol (2 g) magnesium sulphate over 15 min. Q–T interval varies with rate; to calculate the corrected Q–T interval (QT_c):

$QT_c = (QT)/\sqrt{(R-R)} < 0.42$ s

(rule of thumb: if $QT < \frac{1}{2}R-R$ interval then it is not prolonged).

Lucy's ABGs (on 40 per cent O_2) are shown in the table.

pH	7.38 (7.35–7.45)
Po_2 (kPa)	11.2 (> 10.6)
Pco_2 (kPa)	3.4 (4.7–6)
HCO_3^- (mmol/L)	24 (22–28)
BE	−1.2 (±2)

Q List two ABG markers of a *life-threatening* attack　　　　1 mark

1. **Normal or high Pco_2: should normally be low secondary to hyperventilation.**

2. **Respiratory failure, i.e. $Po_2 < 8$ kPa irrespective of O_2 therapy.**

3. **Acidosis: either respiratory or metabolic (caused by lactic acid build-up resulting from increased respiratory effort).**

Q Give two reasons why you would request a chest radiograph　　　1 mark

1. **Exclude a pneumothorax: may be a cause of sudden deterioration in patients with asthma.**

2. **Exclude pneumonia: infective exacerbation.**

❶ Other investigations include FBC (although the WCC is often raised as a result of steroids/stress response in the absence of infection), C-reactive protein (CRP), blood cultures (if pyrexial), sputum cultures and urea and electrolytes (U&Es, e.g. low potassium associated with β_2 agonists or steroid use).

Lucy is diagnosed with a severe asthma attack and is treated appropriately.

Q List two ways in which the effects of treatment can be assessed non-invasively　　　　1 mark

Respiratory

1. Clinically, e.g. respiratory rate, wheeze, ability to complete sentences.

2. Pulse oximetry (Sao_2).

3. PEF.

Lucy's breathing improves and she is transferred to the wards.

Q **What four things should Lucy have before discharge?**   **4 marks**

1. Been on discharge medications for 24 h.

2. Treatment with oral and inhaled steroids in addition to bronchodilators.

3. PEF > 75 per cent best or predicted and < 25 per cent variability.

4. Inhaler technique checked.

5. Management plan agreed using PEF monitoring and symptoms.

6. GP follow-up appointment within 2 working days.

7. Appointment at respiratory clinic within 1 month.

Step 5: oral corticosteroids
Use once daily oral corticosteroids at lowest possible dose
Refer to respiratory clinic

Step 4: persistent poor control
Inhaled corticosteroid up to 2000 µg/day
Consider trials of:
Leukotriene receptor antagonist
Oral theophylline
Oral $β_2$ agonist

Step 3: add-on therapy
Add long acting $β_2$ agonist: if good response continue; if no response stop
If inadequate control increase inhaled corticostreroid to 800 µg/day

Step 2: Regular preventer therapy
Add inhaled corticosteroid: 200–800 µg/day

Step 1: mild, intermittent asthma
Use inhaled short-acting $β_2$ agonist as required

❶ The aims of management of chronic asthma are symptom control, prevention of exacerbations and maximising lung function. Management involves a stepwise approach (see figure).

Total **20 marks**

REFERENCE

British Thoracic Society (BTS). *British Guideline on the Management of Asthma*: **www.brit-thoracic.org.uk**

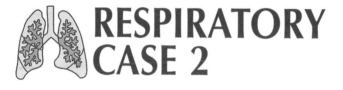# RESPIRATORY CASE 2

Tom, a 73-year-old lifelong smoker with known COPD, is admitted to A&E with severe dyspnoea and cough productive of green sputum. On examination his temperature is 37°C, pulse 95 beats/min, respiratory rate 35/min, he has widespread expiratory wheeze and reduced air entry throughout, and he is cyanosed.

Q **List four differential diagnoses**   2 marks

1. **COPD exacerbation.**

2. **Acute asthma attack**

3. **Pneumonia.**

4. **Acute pulmonary oedema.**

5. **Pulmonary embolism.**

6. **Pneumothorax.**

Q **What four brief questions would you ask about his COPD?**   2 marks

1. **Usual treatments including home nebulisers and oxygen therapy.**

2. **Previous acute episodes and their treatment.**

3. **Normal exercise tolerance.**

4. **Smoking history.**

5. **Any allergies to any medications, e.g. penicillin.**

? QUESTIONS
PAGES
106–108

Respiratory

Q **What is your immediate management?** 3 marks

1. **Controlled O_2 therapy: aim is to keep Sao_2 > 90 per cent without worsening respiratory acidosis/hypercapnia (see below).**

2. **Nebulised bronchodilators, i.e. salbutamol (2.5–5 mg four times daily) and ipratropium bromide (500 μg four times daily).**

3. **Oral steroids: 30 mg prednisolone for 7–14 days (after which it can be stopped abruptly or tapered if previous difficulty coming off steroids; if prolonged treatment will require dose reduction on cessation to avoid a potential addisonian crisis).**

Q **What four non-invasive investigations would you do?** 2 marks

1. **Chest radiograph: exclude pneumonia, pulmonary oedema, pneumothorax.**

2. **ECG: e.g. may show right heart strain (right axis deviation, dominant R waves in V1, right bundle-branch block [RBBB], peaked P waves [P pulmonale]); also to exclude co-morbidities.**

3. **Sputum cultures + sensitivities: identify any infecting organism.**

4. **Pulse oximetry (Sao_2).**

❶ Monitoring PEF in a known COPD patient is not recommended because the magnitude of change is small compared with the variability of the measurement.

❶ Blood tests include FBC (raised WCC may indicate an infective exacerbation), CRP, U&Es, ABGs and blood cultures if pyrexial (though pyrexia is uncommon in COPD exacerbations).

The ABG results (on air) are shown in the table.

pH	7.37 (7.35–7.45)
Po_2 (kPa)	6.9 (> 10.6)
Pco_2 (kPa)	4.2 (4.7–6)
HCO_3^- (mmol/L)	25 (22–28)
BE	−1.2 (±2)

Respiratory

Q What do the ABGs indicate? 2 marks

1. Type I respiratory failure.

❶ The pH and bicarbonate are within normal limits. $Po_2 < 8$ kPa, i.e. respiratory failure, without Pco_2 retention, i.e. type I as opposed to type II.

Q How will these results influence your immediate management? 1 mark

1. As ABGs do not indicate CO_2 retention, increase O_2 aiming for Sao_2 > 92 per cent.

❶ In the presence of type II respiratory failure (i.e. $Pco_2 > 6$ kPa), O_2 therapy should be limited to 24–28 per cent because the respiratory centre is insensitive to CO_2 and respiration is driven by hypoxia. Excessive O_2 therapy may cause life-threatening hypercapnia.

❶ To prevent precipitating or worsening respiratory acidosis, ABGs should be repeated approximately 20 min after each change in O_2 treatment until the patient is stable.

Q List four signs of hypercapnia 2 marks

1. Tachycardia.

2. Bounding pulse.

3. Peripheral vasodilatation.

4. Hand flap.

5. Papilloedema.

6. Confusion.

7. Coma.

❶ Non-invasive ventilation (NIV), e.g. BiPAP (bilevel positive airway pressure), should be considered for any patient with respiratory acidosis/hypercapnia. Worsening respiratory acidosis on treatment is a sensitive indicator of a deteriorating patient and may require admittance to the ICU for invasive ventilation.

Respiratory

The diagnosis is made of infective COPD exacerbation, which is successfully treated with amoxicillin.

Q What two organisms are commonly responsible for COPD exacerbations? 2 marks

1. *Streptococcus pneumoniae.*

2. *Haemophilus influenzae.*

3. *Moraxella catarrhalis.*

❶ Oral antibiotics should be prescribed only if purulent sputum or sputum volume has increased with worsening dyspnoea; typically amoxicillin or erythromycin (if allergic to penicillin) is prescribed. Both antibiotics should be given if the chest radiograph shows pneumonia.

Q On discharge, list four issues to be addressed in collaboration with Tom's GP 2 marks

1. **Smoking cessation.**

2. **Immunisations: flu (annually) and pneumococcal (i.e. *Streptococcus pneumoniae* – once only).**

3. **Compliance with regular inhaled treatment.**

4. **Assessment for home O$_2$.**

❶ The treatment of stable COPD involves short-acting bronchodilators (e.g. salbutamol and/or ipratropium; tiotropium, a long-acting anticholinergic, is also useful) and/or a long-acting β$_2$ agonist (e.g. salmeterol) ± inhaled steroid (fluticasone) if the forced expiratory volume in 1 s (FEV$_1$) < 50 per cent. Mucolytic therapy may also be used if there is chronic productive cough. Maintenance therapy with oral steroids is not recommended. However, some patients may be difficult to wean after a COPD exacerbation; such patients should be managed on the lowest dose possible with osteoporosis prophylaxis.

Respiratory

301

Q List two qualifying criteria for home O$_2$ therapy   **2 marks**

1. **Ex-smoker.**

2. **Po$_2$ < 7.3 kPa (on two separate occasions when COPD is stable, at least 3 weeks apart).**

3. **Po$_2$ < 8 kPa with evidence of secondary polycythaemia, nocturnal hypoxaemia or cor pulmonale.**

❶ To achieve improved survival (50 per cent improvement in 3-year survival), O$_2$ therapy (1–3 L/min) must be given > 15 h/day.

❶ Cor pulmonale is right heart failure secondary to chronic pulmonary hypertension (of which COPD is the most common cause). Characteristics of cor pulmonale include peripheral oedema, raised jugular venous pressure (JVP), right ventricular heave and loud pulmonary second heart sound (see above for ECG changes).

Total   **20 marks**

REFERENCE

British Thoracic Society. *COPD Guidelines*: www.brit-thoracic.org.uk

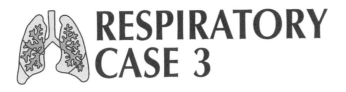

RESPIRATORY CASE 3

Charlotte, a 36-year-old woman, presents to A&E with sudden onset of severe right-sided pleuritic chest pain with associated breathlessness and feeling dizzy. She is normally fit and well, having recently returned from a week's holiday in Florida. She is not on any prescribed medicines except the combined oral contraceptive pill. On examination she has a tender, swollen, right calf.

Q List six risk factors for PE   3 marks

❶ Risk factors are any cause of immobility or hypercoagulability:

1. **Recent surgery, e.g. major abdominal or pelvic surgery, hip or knee replacement.**

2. **Prolonged immobilisation, e.g. plaster cast, bed rest, recent air travel.**

3. **Malignancy, e.g. abdominal, pelvic, advanced metastatic.**

4. **Pregnancy and puerperium.**

5. **Drugs: combined oral contraceptive pill, hormone replacement therapy (HRT).**

6. **Hypercoagulability disorders, i.e. thrombocytosis, polycythaemia, thrombophilia.**

7. **Family history of deep vein thrombosis (DVT)/PE.**

8. **Previous DVT/PE.**

❶ Examples of thrombophilia include anti-phospholipid syndrome (lupus anticoagulant and/or anti-cardiolipin antibody), factor V Leiden (activated protein C resistance), anti-thrombin III deficiency, protein C or S deficiency, and pro-thrombin gene mutation.

QUESTIONS PAGES 109–111

Respiratory

Q **List three differential diagnoses for a tender, swollen calf**   3 marks

1. **DVT.**

2. **Cellulitis: erythema suggests cellultis.**

3. **Ruptured Baker's cyst.**

4. **Trauma.**

5. **Muscle tear.**

6. **Superficial thrombophlebitis.**

❶ Most PEs arise from venous thrombosis in the pelvis or proximal lower limb. However, none of the signs of a DVT (e.g. swollen calf, distended veins, tenderness, increased warmth) is unique to a DVT, which can be reliably confirmed only by Doppler ultrasound examination (if negative but clinical suspicion remains high, use venography).

Q **What six investigations would you do?**   6 marks

1. **FBC: polycythaemia, thrombocytosis.**

2. **Baseline clotting screen: in preparation for anticoagulation.**

3. **D-dimer: see below.**

4. **Chest radiograph: often normal in PE or small effusion; used to exclude pneumothorax.**

5. **ECG: often normal although may show sinus tachycardia, RBBB (e.g. widened QRS complex, RSR [M] pattern in V1), right heart strain (e.g. dominant R waves in V1–3), right axis deviation (positive in III, negative in I); the classic $S_I Q_{III} T_{III}$ (i.e. deep S waves in I, pathological Q waves and inverted T waves in III) is rare.**

6. **ABGs: may show reduced Po_2 and reduced Pco_2 (as a result of hyperventilation).**

7. **Computed tomography pulmonary angiogram (CTPA): able to detect clots down to the fifth order pulmonary arteries.**

8. **Ventilation–perfusion scan: looking for perfusion defects with no corresponding ventilation defects.**

❶ A negative D-dimer can accurately exclude a PE. However, it is raised in infection, malignancy and pregnancy, as well as PE, so it has a low sensitivity. It is therefore recommended only to exclude PE in patients with low-to-moderate probability of PE (scored in relation to such criteria as clinical symptoms of DVT, no alternative diagnosis, immobilisation or recent surgery, previous DVT/PE, malignancy).

❶ If the D-dimer is negative (with a low-to-moderate clinical score) a PE can be reliably excluded (D-dimer should not be performed if the score is high). Otherwise, request a CTPA (older patients, coexisting lung disease) or a ventilation–perfusion scan (younger patients).

❶ Thrombophilia screen is reserved for younger patients with recurrent PEs or a strong family history of DVT/PE. Investigations for occult malignancy are indicated only when it is suspected on clinical examination (including per rectum examination), chest radiograph or routine blood tests.

Charlotte's ECG is shown here.

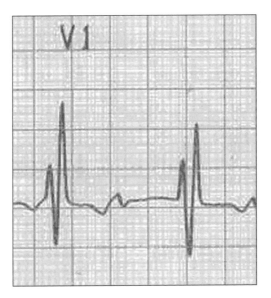

Q What does this ECG show?   **2 marks**

1. **Right bundle branch block (RBBB).**

ⓘ RSR pattern and widened QRS complex and inverted T wave in V1. May also get deep S wave in V6.

The diagnosis of PE secondary to a DVT is made. Charlotte is discharged on a 3-month course of warfarin with a target INR of 2–3 and an anticoagulant card to carry.

Q **What four pieces of general advice would you give to prevent a DVT during a plane flight?** 2 marks

1. **Wear compression stockings.**

2. **Ensure adequate hydration.**

3. **Avoid alcohol during the flight.**

4. **Do not remain seated for long periods – get up and walk around if only to the toilet.**

ⓘ There is no evidence that aspirin is effective at preventing DVT; LMWH are reserved for high risk patients.

Q **What is the mechanism of action of warfarin?** 1 mark

1. **Vitamin K antagonist.**

ⓘ Warfarin inhibits the reductase enzyme responsible for regenerating the active form of vitamin K (needed for the synthesis of factors II, VII, IX and X). Heparin enhances the effects of anti-thrombin III and deactivates factor X (as does low-molecular-weight heparin [LMWH]).

ⓘ The treatment of PE involves O_2, analgesia, TED (thromboembolic deterrent) stockings, LMWH and, in Charlotte's case, stopping the pill. Thrombolysis is reserved for patients with massive PE causing shock. Once the DVT/PE has been confirmed, start warfarin; LMWH should be continued for at least 5 days and to an INR in the therapeutic range (2–3) for ≥ 2 days before it is stopped. This is because, initially, warfarin has a pro-thrombotic effect (proteins C and S are also vitamin K dependent), so the patient needs to be adequately anticoagulated when starting warfarin.

Respiratory

Six weeks later Charlotte is treated for a minor chest infection by her GP with erythromycin (an enzyme inhibitor).

Q **Is she at risk, if so of what and how should this be assessed?**   3 marks

1. **Yes: she is at risk because erythromycin interacts with warfarin. Warfarin is metabolised by hepatic cytochrome P450 enzymes which are inhibited by a number of drugs, including erythromycin.**

2. **Cytochrome P450 inhibition will potentiate the anticoagulant effects of warfarin by preventing its metabolism, increasing the risk of haemorrhage.**

3. **The INR should be monitored more closely and the maintenance dose reduced/omitted if the target INR is exceeded.**

Total   20 marks

REFERENCE

British Thoracic Society. Guidelines on the management of suspected acute pulmonary embolism. *Thorax* 2003;58:470–484: www.brit-thoracic.org.uk

Respiratory

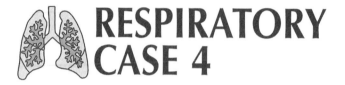# RESPIRATORY
CASE 4

Margaret, a 64-year-old heavy smoker, visits her GP complaining of a 3-month history of cough associated with haemoptysis.

Q **List three respiratory causes of haemoptysis**   3 marks

1. **Acute lower respiratory tract infections.**

2. **Lung cancer.**

3. **Tuberculosis (TB).**

4. **Bronchiectasis: may be a cause of massive haemoptysis.**

5. **Trauma, e.g. inhalation of a foreign body.**

6. **Pulmonary embolism**

❶ Patients who present with haemoptysis should have an urgent chest radiograph to exclude underlying lung cancer.

Q **List two other common presenting lung cancer symptoms**   2 marks

1. **Dyspnoea.**

2. **Chest pain.**

3. **Weight loss.**

4. **Non-resolving pneumonia: patients treated for pneumonia who have persistent chest symptoms/signs or at risk of lung cancer should have a follow-up chest radiograph at 6 weeks.**

? QUESTIONS
PAGES
112–115

❶ Any patient presenting with unexplained or persistent (> 3 weeks) cough, chest/shoulder pain, dyspnoea, weight loss, chest signs, hoarseness (as a result of involvement of recurrent laryngeal nerve), finger clubbing or cervical/supraclavicular lymphadenopathy should also have an urgent chest radiograph.

On examination the only abnormal finding is that she has clubbing.

Q List two cardiac, two respiratory and two GI causes of clubbing   3 marks

Cardiac:

1. **Cyanotic congenital heart disease.**

2. **Subacute bacterial endocarditis.**

Gastrointestinal:

1. **Inflammatory bowel disease (IBD).**

2. **Cirrhosis.**

3. **Malabsorption, e.g. patients with coeliac disease.**

4. **GI lymphoma.**

Respiratory:

1. **Lung cancer.**

2. **Chronic lung suppuration, e.g. cystic fibrosis, bronchiectasis, empyema, abscess.**

3. **Fibrotic lung disease.**

❶ Clubbing is an example of a paraneoplastic syndrome. It occurs in approximately 30 per cent of cases of lung cancer (lung cancer is the most common cause of clubbing).

The GP arranges an urgent chest radiograph. The radiological report notes opacification of the right apex with destruction of the second rib consistent with bronchial carcinoma.

Respiratory

309

Margaret's chest radiograph is shown here.

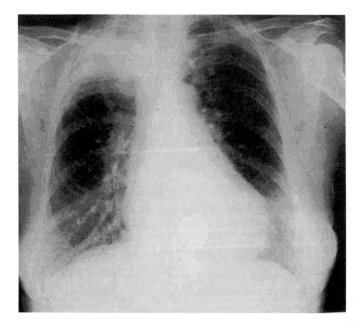

Q What is this type of lung tumour called?   1 mark

1. Pancoast's tumour.

❶ Pancoast's tumour refers to a lung tumour in the apex of the lung. It may cause rib erosion, involve the brachial plexus, causing pain down the medial aspect of the arm, or involve the sympathetic chain, causing Horner's syndrome.

Q List four signs of Horner's syndrome   2 marks

1. Ptosis: drooping of upper eyelid.

2. Miosis: constricted pupil caused by unopposed parasympathetic innervation.

3. Enophthalmos: sunken eye.

4. Ipsilateral loss of facial sweating.

❶ Lung cancer complications can be classified as local, e.g. Horner's syndrome, metastatic (spread to liver, bone, brain) and paraneoplastic syndromes (caused by tumour secretory products).

❶ Other local complications are: superior vena caval obstruction causing early morning headache; puffy face and neck (collar feels tight); distended, non-pulsatile jugular vein; and dilated veins on the chest wall. The obstruction may be relieved by radiotherapy ± stenting of the vein.

❶ Other examples of paraneoplastic syndromes include Eaton–Lambert syndrome (proximal myopathy), ectopic ACTH (adrenocorticotrophic hormone) and hypertrophic pulmonary osteoarthropathy (HPOA), which causes joint stiffness and severe pain in the wrists and ankles; radiographs show subperiosteal new bone formation, often described as an 'onion-skin' appearance. Symptoms improve when the primary tumour is removed.

Q List four causes of round lesions on the lung on a chest radiograph   2 marks

1. **Primary lung tumours: most lung tumours are bronchial carcinomas that can be classified as small cell carcinoma and non-small cell carcinoma (further divided into squamous cell, large cell and adenocarcinoma). Rarer forms of lung tumours include bronchioloalveolar cell carcinoma.**

2. **Secondary lung tumours, e.g. spread from kidney, testis, breast, bone, choriocarcinoma or GI tract (usually multiple).**

3. **'Round pneumonia'.**

4. **Abscess (usually with air–fluid level).**

5. **Cyst, e.g. hydatid.**

6. **Foreign body.**

7. **Granuloma (i.e. nodular accumulation of macrophages), e.g. TB, sarcoidosis.**

8. **Rheumatoid nodule.**

Margaret is seen the following week as an outpatient at the respiratory clinic.

Respiratory

Q **What two investigations would you arrange to confirm lung cancer?** 2 marks

1. **Bronchoscopy: to obtain biopsy for histological diagnosis. Patients require pulmonary function tests and lateral chest radiograph in preparation.**

2. **Computed tomography (CT) of the thorax (plus upper abdomen): to stage the tumour.**

3. **CT-guided biopsy (for peripheral lesions).**

❶ Sputum for cytology is an insensitive test and not routinely performed.

❶ Staging is important for treatment and prognosis. Non-small cell carcinoma is staged using the TNM (tumour, node, metastasis) system; small cell carcinoma, which has usually metastasised at presentation, is staged as limited or extensive. Increasingly, positron emission tomography (PET) is used for staging (detects increased uptake of labelled glucose by cancer cells).

❶ Blood tests include liver function tests (bronchial carcinoma may metastasise to the liver), bone profile (may metastasise to the bone causing ↑ Ca^{2+} and ↑ ALP) and U&Es (e.g. hyponatraemia caused by the syndrome of inappropriate antidiuretic hormone secretion [SIADH] – an example of a paraneoplastic syndrome).

From these tests a diagnosis of inoperable squamous cell bronchial carcinoma is confirmed. Three months later Margaret is admitted with unremitting back pain causing night-time waking. A lateral spinal radiograph confirms secondary deposits in the thoracic vertebrae. She is treated with radiotherapy and opiate analgesia. Her bone profile results are shown in the table.

Adjusted Ca^{2+} (mmol/L)	3.7 (normal range 2.12–2.65)
PO_4^{3-} (mmol/L)	1.4 (normal range 0.8–1.45)
ALP (IU)	190 (normal range 30–150)

Q List four causes of raised serum calcium   4 marks

1. **Malignant disease: may be caused by bony metastases (common primary tumours are of the lung, breast, thyroid, prostate, oesophagus, kidney, myeloma) or secretion of PTH-related protein (PTH-rp).**

2. **Excessive PTH secretion: may be the result of primary or tertiary hyperparathyroidism. The primary form is caused by parathyroid hyperplasia, adenoma or carcinoma, and usually causes mild hypercalcaemia. The secondary form is compensatory parathyroid hypertrophy in response to chronic hypocalcaemia (e.g. in renal failure); calcium levels are low or normal. The tertiary form is the result of prolonged stimulation of the parathyroid in long-standing hypocalcaemia, so that PTH release is no longer under feedback control of calcium.**

3. **Hyperthyroidism.**

4. **Excessive calcium intake.**

5. **Excessive vitamin D intake.**

6. **Drugs, e.g. thiazides (calcium-sparing diuretics).**

7. **Sarcoidosis (producing excess vitamin D).**

❶ More than 90 per cent of cases of hypercalcaemia are caused by malignancy or hyperparathyroidism.

Q How would you treat Margaret's hypercalcaemia?   1 mark

❶ Acute hypercalcaemia often presents with dehydration as a result of vomiting and polyuria, severe abdominal pain and constipation, and confusion. If the patient is symptomatic or serum $Ca^{2+} > 3.5$ mmol/L, reduce hypercalcaemia as follows:

1. **Rehydrate with intravenous saline (0.9 per cent) 4–6 L/day to correct any hypovolaemia from vomiting and polyuria.**

2. **Bisphosphonates: inhibit osteoclast activity, thereby reducing bone resorption.**

Respiratory

❶ The treatment of lung cancer includes surgery (lobectomy or pneumonectomy), radiotherapy and/or chemotherapy. For non-small cell carcinoma chemotherapy offers very little survival benefit; small cell carcinoma is very sensitive to chemotherapy (increasing median survival from 3 months to 12–18 months).

Total   **20 marks**

REFERENCE

National Institute for Health and Clinical Excellence (NICE). *The Diagnosis and Treatment of Lung Cancer*, 2005: www.nice.org.uk

Respiratory

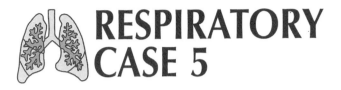

RESPIRATORY
CASE 5

John, a 72 year old insulin dependent diabetic, attends his GP with a 3-day history of cough, dyspnoea and general malaise. He is prescribed amoxicillin but continues to deteriorate and is admitted to hospital the following day. John's chest radiograph is shown here.

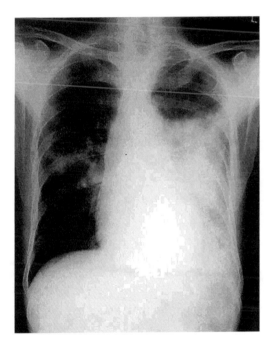

Q What is your diagnosis?   **1 mark**

1. Left lower lobe pneumonia.

❶ Loss of the left hemidiaphragm and preservation of the left heart border indicate that the pneumonia is in the left lower lobe.

QUESTIONS
PAGES
116–118

❶ Involvement of only one lobe is a good prognostic indicator; conversely bilateral or multilobe pneumonia on chest radiograph indicates severe pneumonia (see below).

Q List two poor prognostic features in the history above   2 marks

1. Age 72 years.

2. Diabetes.

❶ Age > 50 years and coexisting chronic disease are associated with a poor prognosis. Failure to respond to treatment would also represent a poor prognostic sign, although in this case John has received only a short course of oral antibiotics. Cough and dyspnoea are not sensitive markers of the severity of pneumonia.

A full examination is performed and appropriate investigations undertaken.

Q List three findings on *examination* that would indicate severe pneumonia   3 marks

1. (New) confusion, i.e. delirium, e.g. score of < 8/10 on Abbreviated Mental Test Score (AMTS).

2. Tachypnoea, i.e. respiratory rate > 30/min.

3. Hypotension, i.e. systolic BP < 90 mmHg or diastolic BP < 60 mmHg.

Q List three findings on *investigation* that would indicate severe pneumonia   3 marks

1. Po_2 < 8 kPa (or Sao_2 < 92 per cent) regardless of inspired oxygen concentration.

2. Raised urea, i.e. > 7 mmol/L.

3. WCC > 20 × 10^9/L (leukocytosis) or < 4 × 10^9/L (leukopenia).

4. Positive blood culture.

❶ Appropriate investigations include FBC, CRP, U&Es, LFTs, blood cultures, ABGs (if Sao_2 < 92 per cent) and sputum for MC&S; in severe cases screen for atypical organisms (see below).

❶ The British Thoracic Society (BTS) CURB-65 score is a simple tool for assessing severity, i.e. two or more of the following indicate severe pneumonia:

• Confusion < 8/10 AMTS

• Urea >7 mmol/L

• Respiratory rate > 30/min

• BP: systolic < 90 mmHg or diastolic < 60 mmHg

• Age > 65 years.

❶ Management of pneumonia is based on its severity. If not severe treat with oral antibiotics, e.g. amoxicillin 500 mg three times daily and clarithromycin 500 mg twice daily. If severe treat with intravenous antibiotics, e.g. either co-amoxiclav 1.2 g three times daily or cefuroxime 1.5 g three times daily with clarithromycin 500 mg twice daily.

John is diagnosed with severe pneumonia and treated with intravenous cefuroxime and clarithromycin (to cover atypical organisms).

Q **List three causes of 'atypical' pneumonia**   3 marks

1. *Mycoplasma pneumoniae*: **tends to affect young adults; it occurs in epidemics every 3–4 years.**

2. *Legionella pneumophila*: **outbreaks are usually associated with contaminated showers, or water-cooling or air-conditioning systems.**

3. *Coxiella burnetii* **(Q fever).**

4. *Chlamydia* **species, e.g.** *C. psittaci, C. pneumoniae.*

❶ It is important in the history to enquire about any pet birds *(C. psittaci)* or recent stay in a hotel *(Legionella).*

Respiratory

317

❶ Atypical infections are 'atypical' because they do not respond to penicillin (treat with macrolides, e.g. erythromycin, clarithromycin) and cause general (e.g. diarrhoea) as well as respiratory symptoms.

❶ In patients with severe pneumonia (or suspicion of atypical pneumonia) blood should be sent for atypical serology (i.e. specific antibodies against atypical organisms) and urine screened for legionella antigen (can also screen for pneumococcal antigen).

Microbiology call the ward to report Gram-positive cocci in John's blood while awaiting culture and sensitivity.

Q **What is the most likely cause of John's pneumonia and how can this be prevented?** 2 marks

1. *Streptococcus pneumoniae* **is a Gram-positive (i.e. stains purple) coccus and is the most common cause of pneumonia, accounting for 60–75 per cent of cases; it responds to penicillins.**

2. **Pneumococcal immunisation: should be offered to all those with a chronic illness, e.g. patients with diabetes.**

❶ Other common causes of community-acquired pneumonia include *Mycoplasma pneumoniae* (5–15 per cent – intracellular organism that does not Gram stain) and *Haemophilus influenzae* (5 per cent – Gram negative). *Staphylococcus aureus* is also a Gram-positive coccus but is not a common cause of pneumonia; typically affects intravenous drug users (IVDUs).

Q **List six parameters used to assess treatment progress** 3 marks

1. **Heart rate.**

2. **Respiratory rate.**

3. **Blood pressure.**

4. **Temperature.**

5. **Sao_2 (or O_2 requirements necessary to maintain adequate Sao_2).**

6. **Mental status.**

7. **CRP: this is a sensitive marker of treatment progress.**

8. **WCC.**

❶ In patients not progressing satisfactorily, the chest radiograph should be repeated to look for complications.

John fails to make good progress and clinical examination reveals reduced breath sounds at the right base. His chest radiograph is repeated, which shows a right pleural effusion.

Q **What is the most likely complication?**   1 mark

1. **Empyema.**

❶ Empyema refers to pus in the pleural space. The fluid should be tapped and sent for pH analysis. If the pH < 7.2 the effusion should be treated as an empyema (see below). Untreated, extensive fibrosis occurs in the pleural cavity, weight loss and clubbing develop, and the mortality rate is high.

❶ Other complications of pneumonia that may be seen on a chest radiograph include pleural effusion and lung abscess (cavitating area of localised suppurative [pus-forming] infection – appears as a fluid-filled cavity).

Q **How should this be treated?**   2 marks

1. **Tube drainage: intrapleural fibrinolytic, e.g. streptokinase is given twice daily into the drain to liquefy pus and aid drainage.**

2. **High-dose intravenous antibiotics.**

Total   20 marks

REFERENCE

British Thoracic Society. *Guidelines on the Management of Community Acquired Pneumonia in Adults*, 2004: www.brit-thoracic.org.uk

Respiratory

RHEUMATOLOGY
CASES: ANSWERS

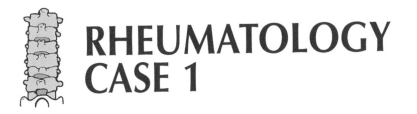

RHEUMATOLOGY CASE 1

Hayley, a 36-year-old woman, attends her GP with a 2-month history of stiff, painful, swollen hands associated with general malaise.

Q List four *inflammatory* causes of *polyarthropathy* 　　　　4 marks

1. **Rheumatoid arthritis (RA): systemic disease causing a symmetrical polyarthritis.**

2. **Seronegative arthropathy (arthritis associated with psoriasis, inflammatory bowel disease and ankylosing spondylitis)**

3. **Reactive arthritis: arthritis following infection, e.g. post-dysentery or non-gonococcal urethritis (NGU).**

4. **Arthritis associated with viral illness, e.g. parvovirus or mumps.**

5. **Connective tissue disorders, e.g. SLE, Sjögren's syndrome.**

6. **Lyme disease: tick-borne infection caused by *Borrelia burgdorferi*.**

Examination of Hayley's hands and wrists shows changes characteristic of rheumatoid arthritis.

Q Give eight features of RA in the hands and wrists on examination　4 marks

1. **Boggy swelling (synovitis) of proximal small joints of hands (metacarpophalangeal [MCP], proximal interphalangeal [PIP]).**

2. **Tender, erythematous, hot joints.**

3. **Loss of 'valleys' around the knuckles on making a fist: as a result of MCP joint swelling.**

4. **Sausage-shaped fingers (spindling): as a result of soft tissue swelling.**

5. **Wasting of small muscles of the hand.**

6. **Swan-neck deformity: fixed hyperextension of PIP joint and flexion of DIP (distal interphalangeal) joint.**

7. **Boutonnière (or button-hole) deformity: fixed flexion of PIP joint.**

8. **Z deformity of the thumb.**

9. **Finger drop: caused by rupture of finger extensor tendons (after wrist subluxation).**

10. **Subluxation of the wrist.**

11. **Prominent radial head (piano key).**

12. **Loss of function.**

13. **Symmetrical changes, i.e. involvement of both hands.**

❶ RA is a systemic inflammatory disorder that affects predominantly women (3:1 sex ratio) and can occur at any age. It typically presents with pain, stiffness and swelling of the proximal small joints of the hands and feet.

❶ Other less common presentations of RA include monoarthritis (a single swollen joint) or palindromic arthritis (joint swelling that occurs intermittently, lasting just a few days at a time).

Hayley is sent for a radiograph of her hands.

Q Give four radiological changes in the hands in RA   **2 marks**

❶ Early changes:

1. **Soft tissue swelling.**

2. **Juxta-articular osteopenia.**

3. **Loss of joint space.**

Rheumatology

❶ Late changes:

1. **Bony erosions at the joint margins.**

2. **Subluxation and dislocation of joints.**

3. **Carpal bone destruction.**

❶ Other investigations include: FBC (normochromic anaemia, raised WCC), raised ESR and/or CRP, rheumatoid factor (RF) and anti-nuclear antibody (ANA – positive in 30 per cent of patients).

❶ Rheumatoid factors are autoantibodies directed at antibodies, e.g. anti-IgG IgM. Although often negative at the start of RA, they eventually become positive in 70–80 per cent of patients. However, RFs are not diagnostic of RA because they are present in up to 10 per cent of the general population, although they are prognostic; patients with a positive RF usually follow a more aggressive disease course. 'Seronegative' RA (and seronegative arthritides) refers to patients with arthropathy but with no RFs detectable in the blood. These individuals tend to have milder joint disease.

Q **List four criteria on history, examination and investigation used to diagnose RA**   **4 marks**

1. **Morning stiffness > 1 h (for ≥ 6 weeks).**

2. **Arthritis of three or more joints (for ≥ 6 weeks).**

3. **Arthritis of hand and wrist joints (for ≥ 6 weeks).**

4. **Symmetrical arthritis (for ≥ 6 weeks).**

5. **Rheumatoid nodules (most common at sites of pressure, e.g. extensor surfaces of forearm).**

6. **RF seropositivity.**

7. **Typical radiological changes.**

❶ RA is diagnosed on the basis of four or more positive criteria.

Q List four features associated with a poor prognosis 2 marks

1. **Female sex.**

2. **Multiple joint involvement.**

3. **Early functional disability.**

4. **Early radiological changes.**

5. **Extra-articular features.**

6. **Insidious onset.**

7. **HLA-DR4 positive.**

8. **High titres of RF.**

❶ RA is a systemic disease affecting many organs: eyes (Sjögren's syndrome [dry eyes], scleritis), cardiovascular system (pericarditis, pericardial effusions, Raynaud's phenomenon), respiratory system (pleural effusions, nodules and Caplan's syndrome, fibrosing alveolitis, bronchiectasis), skin (ulcers, nodules, vasculitis, pyoderma grangrenosum), nervous system (carpal tunnel syndrome, peripheral neuropathy, mononeuritis multiplex, cervical myelopathy), Felty's syndrome (splenomegaly and neutropenia associated with infections, anaemia, thrombocytopenia and lymphadenopathy), kidneys (renal failure) and secondary systemic amyloidosis.

Hayley is diagnosed with RA and started on NSAIDs by her GP. She is also referred to a rheumatologist for consideration of a DMARD.

Q Name two DMARDs and two side effects associated with each 4 marks

Rheumatology

DMARD	Associated side effects
Methotrexate	Hepatotoxicity (rarely fatal hepatitis), bone marrow suppression, pulmonary fibrosis, mucositis, e.g. mouth ulcers
Sulfasalazine	Bone marrow suppression, oligospermia, skin rash, gastrointestinal (GI) side effects (e.g. nausea), hepatotoxicity
Leflunomide	Bone marrow suppression, GI side effects, hypertension
Penicillamine	Skin rash, proteinuria (may progress to renal failure), GI side effects (metallic taste, nausea)
Gold	Proteinuria (may progress to renal failure), skin rash, blood dyscrasia, GI side effects (e.g. diarrhoea)
Anti-malarials, e.g. hydroxychloroquine and chloroquine	Corneal deposits, retinopathy
Azathioprine	Bone marrow suppression, hepatotoxicity, GI side effects (e.g. nausea)
Cyclophosphamide	Bone marrow suppression, carcinogenesis, pulmonary toxicity, GI side effects (e.g. nausea), cardiac toxicity (e.g. heart failure, arrhythmias)
Tumour necrosis factor α inhibitors, e.g. infliximab, etanercept	Infections, e.g. TB, septicaemia, worsening heart failure, injection site reactions and blood dyscrasias

❶ Treatment of RA includes patient education, physical therapy, splints, surgery and pharmacological treatments. Pharmacological treatments include simple analgesia, NSAIDs, corticosteroids (both orally and intra-articular injections; used for acute exacerbations and to control symptoms while DMARDs are being introduced) and DMARDs, including the newer biological agents, e.g. tumour necrosis factor α (TNF-α) inhibitors.

❶ DMARDs suppress the disease process in RA (as evidenced by reduction in symptoms, joint swelling, fall in ESR/CRP and retardation in radiological joint damage), typically through cytokine inhibition, although, unlike NSAIDs, they take several months for full response. They are typically prescribed in patients with poor prognostic features (see above). Patients are initially prescribed either methotrexate or sulfasalazine; patients with a poor response to initial therapy are changed to an alternative DMARD or are started on combination DMARD therapy. Early aggressive treatment slows (and in some individuals may even halt) disease progression.

Rheumatology

❶ TNF-α inhibitors have been recommended by the National Institute for Health and Clinical Excellence (NICE) for highly active RA when there has been a failure to respond to two DMARDs. Prescribing and monitoring of these agents should be done by a rheumatologist and they should be withdrawn after 3 months if there is no response to treatment or serious side effects develop. They are very expensive (approximately £10 000/year).

Total **20 marks**

RHEUMATOLOGY CASE 2

Julie is a 28-year-old woman with a past history of depression. She attends her GP complaining of fatigue and joint pains for the last 2 months. On examination she has a butterfly facial rash.

Q How else may SLE present?   4 marks

1. **Fever.**

2. **Weight loss.**

3. **Mouth ulcers.**

4. **Hair loss (alopecia).**

5. **Chest pain (pleuritic).**

6. **Leg swelling (oedema).**

7. **Limb weakness (stroke).**

8. **Seizures.**

9. **Depression or psychosis.**

10. **Raynaud's phenomenon.**

ⓘ SLE is an autoimmune disease that can affect almost any system in the body. It occurs more commonly in females (particularly those who are African–Caribbean), typically presenting in early adult life (although it can present at any age – neonates or very elderly people). Its presenting symptoms are highly variable and mild cases may present with only arthralgia and fatigue. Therefore always consider SLE in your differential in any woman who presents with inflammatory arthritis.

QUESTIONS PAGES 124–125

Rheumatology

ⓘ Numerous drugs are associated with causing a lupus-like syndrome, e.g. isoniazid, hydralazine. Drug lupus typically affects the skin and lungs; kidney and central nervous system (CNS) involvement is rare. The symptoms resolve once the drug is stopped.

Q List eight investigations that you would request   **8 marks**

1. **FBC: leukopenia, lymphopenia, thrombocytopenia.**

2. **U&Es: renal impairment.**

3. **ESR: elevated.**

4. **CRP: usually normal in SLE.**

5. **Autoantibody screen, e.g. ANA, double-stranded (anti ds) DNA, anti-Sm.**

6. **Serum complement levels: reduced C3 and C4 levels (as a result of active consumption).**

7. **Urinalysis: proteinuria, red blood cell (RBC) casts.**

8. **ECG: pericarditis, e.g. first-degree heart block.**

9. **Chest radiograph, e.g. pleural effusion.**

10. **Joint radiographs: erosive changes are not seen in SLE, and would be more suggestive of RA.**

ⓘ SLE is diagnosed on the basis of four or more of the following *clinical* and *laboratory* criteria:

- Malar (butterfly) rash

- Discoid rash: erythematous raised patches that eventually progress to areas of scarring; discoid lupus is restricted to the skin with no systemic involvement

- Skin photosensitivity

- Oral ulcers (oral or nasopharyngeal)

- Arthritis: radiologically the joints appear normal, i.e. non-erosive

- Serositis: pleuritis (e.g. pleuritic chest pain), pleural effusion, pericarditis

- Renal involvement: proteinuria 3+, cellular casts, e.g. RBC casts

Rheumatology

- Neurological disorder: seizures, psychosis

- Haematological disorder: anaemia, leukopenia, thrombocytopenia, lymphopenia

- Immunological disorder: anti-ds DNA antibody; anti-Sm antibody, anti-phospholipid antibodies, false-positive syphilis test

- ANA positive.

❶ The clinical features of SLE are caused by autoantibodies against a range of antigens, e.g. ANA antibodies occur in 95 per cent of SLE cases although they are also present in other autoimmune diseases (e.g. RA, scleroderma) so they are not diagnostic. Anti-ds DNA and anti-Sm are the SLE-specific antibodies occurring in approximately 80 per cent and 30 per cent of cases, respectively.

❶ Complement levels, ESR and anti-ds DNA antibodies can be used to monitor disease activity. CRP is very useful in differentiating an SLE flare-up from infection because CRP is usually normal in a flare but raised in infection. Infection, caused by both the disease itself and immunosuppressants, is a major cause of early mortality.

Julie's blood tests show a strongly positive ANA titre. She also has a raised ESR. Urinalysis shows 3+ proteinuria.

Q **What is the likely cause of Julie's proteinuria?**   **1 mark**

1. **Lupus nephritis: SLE is a cause of glomerulonephritis.**

❶ Clinical manifestations of lupus nephritis vary from hypertension and nephrotic syndrome (proteinuria, hypoalbuminaemia, hypercholesterolaemia and oedema) to acute renal failure.

❶ Renal disease is the leading cause of early mortality in patients with SLE. Severe renal disease often requires high-dose immunosuppression (e.g. intravenous cyclophosphamide) to control the disease. In long-standing SLE the main cause of mortality is cardiovascular disease (CVD) resulting from accelerated atherosclerosis.

Q **List three treatment options for Julie's joint symptoms**   **3 marks**

Rheumatology

331

1. **NSAIDs: use with caution if renal disease.**

2. **Anti-malarials (hydroxychloroquine): also used for skin disease.**

3. **Oral corticosteroids (low dose).**

4. **Intra-articular steroid injection.**

5. **Physiotherapy.**

❶ SLE is a relapsing and remitting disease. Typically the nature of the disease becomes established in the first 5 years or so; if no significant problems have occurred during this time they are unlikely to do so. Drug therapy should be used only in active flare-ups; there is no benefit of treatment in remission. High-dose oral prednisolone ± steroid-sparing agent (e.g. azathioprine) are used for severe flare-ups with cyclophosphamide reserved for severe disease, e.g. CNS, kidneys, blood dyscrasias.

Two years later Julie is doing well, and speaks to her GP about the possibility of becoming pregnant.

Q **What are the potential problems that Julie might face during her pregnancy?**   4 marks

1. **Flare-up of her SLE.**

2. **Pre-eclampsia.**

3. **Miscarriage.**

4. **Pre-term birth.**

5. **Intrauterine growth retardation.**

6. **Venous thromboembolism (deep vein thrombosis [DVT] or pulmonary embolism [PE]).**

7. **Congenital heart block affecting her baby.**

❶ SLE is a condition that is exacerbated by the presence of female sex hormones. This explains its increased frequency in women, and also why it often presents or flares up during pregnancy. In patients with SLE the presence of certain antibodies (anti-Ro and anti-La antibodies) that cross the placenta can lead to neonatal cardiac conduction defects. It is important to screen for these antibodies in women with known SLE who are considering pregnancy.

ⓘ SLE is associated with anti-phospholipid (APL) syndrome which is characterised by venous and arterial thromboembolism (causing PE, strokes), recurrent miscarriages, thrombocytopenia and livedo reticularis (a brown 'net-like' rash occurring over the lower limbs). It is associated with lupus anticoagulant and anti-cardiolipin antibodies. Paradoxically the activated partial thromboplastin time (APTT) is often elevated (which would normally suggest a tendency towards bleeding rather than clotting); this occurs because these antibodies, which in-vivo cause a thrombotic tendency, interfere with the in-vitro APTT test.

Total   **20 marks**

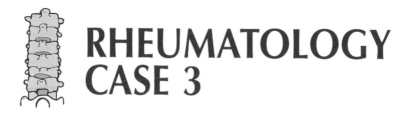

RHEUMATOLOGY CASE 3

Mabel, a 78-year-old woman, attends her GP complaining of pain and stiffness affecting her shoulder, neck and hips. She is unable to sleep at night because of the pain, and has great difficulty in getting out of bed and dressing in the mornings.

Q What blood test would confirm the likely diagnosis of PMR?　　3 marks

1. **ESR: typically > 30 mm/h. Creatine kinase (CK) is normal (although raised in polymyositis).**

ⓘ PMR is a relatively common condition that occurs almost exclusively in people over the age of 60. It is characterised by hip and shoulder girdle stiffness, which is worse in the mornings and eases gradually with activity. The ESR is typically high, and treatment with oral corticosteroids confirms the diagnosis by rapidly relieving the symptoms (symptoms that do not resolve should prompt investigation for an alternative diagnosis).

ⓘ Another important cause of a raised ESR in elderly people is multiple myeloma. This is a malignant disease of plasma cells. It usually presents with anaemia, hypercalcaemia, pathological fractures and renal failure.

Mabel's GP prescribes prednisolone 15 mg daily. However, she decides not to collect the prescription because she has fears about taking steroids. Two weeks later she represents complaining of headache, jaw ache while eating and scalp tenderness when combing her hair.

Q What would be your next steps in management?　　3 marks

1. **Start high-dose prednisolone (60–100 mg daily).**

2. **Refer urgently to an ophthalmologist.**

QUESTIONS
PAGES
126–128

3. **Arrange a temporal artery biopsy: this should be done within 7 days of starting steroids.**

❶ Temporal arteritis (or giant cell arteritis) is part of the clinical spectrum of PMR. It may cause amaurosis fugax or blindness in one eye. Once one eye is affected, the other eye usually follows within days unless appropriate treatment is started.

Q **What steps could have been taken to encourage Mabel to comply with her initial treatment?**   3 marks

1. **Careful explanation of the potential complications of PMR.**

2. **Asking Mabel to feed back what she understood from your explanation.**

3. **Discussing the potential benefits and risks of steroid treatment.**

4. **Specifically asking about fears and concerns about steroids .**

5. **Correcting any misconceptions that she may have about steroids.**

6. **Arranging for a follow-up visit with a doctor or specialist nurse.**

❶ Poor compliance with medications is a major issue in all age groups, but especially elderly people. This is rarely the fault of the patient, but rather a failing on the part of the medical team. Provision of written information about conditions as well as multidisciplinary team input (pharmacists, nurses, etc.) are important steps in managing the elderly patient.

Q **Give eight complications of long-term oral steroid treatment**   4 marks

1. **Impaired glucose tolerance (may progress to diabetes mellitus).**

2. **Mental disturbance, e.g. euphoria, agitation or depression.**

3. **Osteoporosis (especially a risk in postmenopausal women).**

4. **Avascular necrosis of the femoral neck.**

5. **Cushing's syndrome: easy bruising, moon face, buffalo hump, striae.**

6. **Wasting and thinning of the skin.**

7. **Muscle wasting (proximal myopathy).**

8. **Hypertension.**

Rheumatology

9. **Dyspepsia (may also cause peptic ulcer disease).**

10. **Cataracts.**

11. **Immunosuppression increasing risk of infections.**

❶ Prolonged use of corticosteroids may also cause suppression of the hypothalamus–pituitary–adrenal (HPA) axis. Acute adrenal insufficiency (addisonian crisis) may develop if steroids are withdrawn too quickly or during physiological stress (e.g. surgery, trauma or illness). Therefore, in prolonged steroid treatment, i.e. > 3 weeks, steroids should be withdrawn slowly (to allow the HPA axis to recover) and patients should carry a steroid treatment warning card.

Mabel agrees to start her steroid therapy, and has a rapid improvement in symptoms. She is advised that she is going to need to remain on steroid therapy for 12–18 months at least.

Q **What steps can be taken to reduce her risk of an osteoporotic fracture?**   **5 marks**

1. **Increased dietary intake of calcium, e.g. dairy products.**

2. **Increased level of physical exercise.**

3. **Stop smoking.**

4. **Adequate, safe sunshine exposure.**

5. **Oral calcium and vitamin D supplementation.**

6. **Bisphosphonate therapy: inhibit osteoclast activity, thereby preventing bone resorption.**

❶ The diagnosis of osteoporosis can be confirmed by a DEXA (dual X-ray absorptiometry) scan, which quantifies bone density at the proximal femur and spine, although anyone over the age of 65 who is being started on long-term oral steroids or any postmenopausal woman who has suffered a low trauma fracture should be treated without a prior DEXA scan.

❶ Other risk factors for osteoporosis include smoking, alcohol, low body mass index, postmenopausal, prolonged immobility and malabsorption (e.g. coeliac disease).

ⓘ Osteomalacia has the same radiological appearance as osteoporosis (reduced bone density), and is very common in the elderly population, causing bone or muscle pain. It is therefore an important diagnosis to exclude: reduced serum vitamin D and raised ALP (indicating increased osteoblast activity) and PTH (secondary hyperparathyroidism). Treatment is calcium and vitamin D therapy.

Mabel is commenced on a once-weekly oral bisphosphonate.

Q **What is the major potential adverse effect of bisphosphonate therapy?** 2 marks

1. **Oesophageal and gastric ulceration.**

ⓘ Some individuals are unable to tolerate oral bisphosphonates, in which case intravenous preparations can be administered (e.g. pamidronate every 3 months). In patients in whom bisphosphonates are contraindicated, or who do not respond, e.g. further fractures, or who cannot tolerate them, use strontium (which increases bone formation and decreases bone resorption).

Total **20 marks**

INDEX

*This index covers the answer section only. Page numbers in **bold** indicate the main subject of each case.*